Migrant Health Professionals and the Global Labour Market

This book offers a fresh perspective on gender debates in Nepal and analyses how the international migration of the first generation of professional female Nepali nurses has been a catalyst for social change.

With unprecedented access to study participants in Nepal (the source country), following them and their networks in the UK (the destination country), this ethnographic study explores Nepali nurses' migration journeys, relocation experiences, and their international migration 'dreams' and aspirations. It illustrates how migrant nurses strive to manage social and professional difficulties as they work towards achieving their ultimate migration aims. The book shows that nursing shortages and international nurse migration are issues of gender, on a global scale, and that the current trend of privatisation in health systems makes the labour market vulnerable, and stimulates international migration of health professionals. Arguing that international nurse migration is an integral part of the globalisation of health, the author highlights key policy strategies that are useful for global nursing and health workforce management.

A well-informed and much-needed study of nurse migration in the global healthcare market, this book will be of interest to professionals and academics working in nursing studies, health and social care studies, gender and international migration studies, and global health studies, as well as South Asian studies.

Radha Adhikari is a Nepali nurse and a Research Associate at the Centre for South Asian Studies, University of Edinburgh, UK.

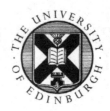

Routledge/Edinburgh South Asian Studies Series

Series Editor:
Crispin Bates and the Editorial Committee of the Centre for South Asian Studies, Edinburgh University, UK.

The *Routledge/Edinburgh South Asian Studies Series* is published in association with the Centre for South Asian Studies, Edinburgh University – one of the leading centres for South Asian Studies in the UK with a strong interdisciplinary focus. This series presents research monographs and high-quality edited volumes as well as textbooks on topics concerning the Indian subcontinent from the modern period to contemporary times. It aims to advance understanding of the key issues in the study of South Asia, and contributions include works by experts in the social sciences and the humanities. In accordance with the academic traditions of Edinburgh, we particularly welcome submissions which emphasise the social in South Asian history, politics, sociology and anthropology, based upon thick description of empirical reality, generalised to provide original and broadly applicable conclusions.

The series welcomes new submissions from young researchers as well as established scholars working on South Asia, from any disciplinary perspective.

Provincial Globalization in India
Transregional Mobilities and Development Politics
Edited by Carol Upadhya, Mario Rutten and Leah Koskimak

Global Health Governance and Commercialisation in India
Actors, Institutions and the Dialectics of Global and Local
Edited by Anuj Kapilashrami and Rama V. Baru

Space, Utopia and Indian Decolonization
Literary Pre-Figurations of the Postcolony
Sandeep Banerjee

Migrant Health Professionals and the Global Labour Market
The dreams and traps of Nepali nurses
Radha Adhikari

For a full list of titles, please see: www.routledge.com/asianstudies/series/RESAS

Migrant Health Professionals and the Global Labour Market

The Dreams and Traps of Nepali Nurses

Radha Adhikari

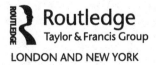
Routledge
Taylor & Francis Group

LONDON AND NEW YORK

First published 2020
by Routledge
2 Park Square, Milton Park, Abingdon, Oxon OX14 4RN

and by Routledge
605 Third Avenue, New York, NY 10017

First issued in paperback 2022

Routledge is an imprint of the Taylor & Francis Group, an informa business

Publisher's Note
The publisher has gone to great lengths to ensure the quality of this reprint but points out that some imperfections in the original copies may be apparent.

British Library Cataloguing in Publication Data
A catalogue record for this book is available from the British Library

Library of Congress Cataloging-in-Publication Data
Names: Adhikari, Radha, author.
Title: Migrant health professionals and the global labour
market : the dreams and traps of Nepali nurses / Radha Adhikari.
Description: 1. | New York : Routledge, 2019. |
Series: Routledge/Edinburgh South Asian studies series |
Includes bibliographical references and index.
Identifiers: LCCN 2019032547 (print) | LCCN 2019032548 (ebook) |
ISBN 9780367344252 (hardback) | ISBN 9780429325731 (ebook) |
ISBN 9781000729689 (adobe pdf) | ISBN 9781000729832 (mobi) |
ISBN 9781000729986 (epub)
Subjects: LCSH: Medical personnel, Foreign. | Nursing--Nepal. |
Emigration and immigration. | Brain drain. | Labor market.
Classification: LCC R697.F6 A34 2019 (print) |
LCC R697.F6 (ebook) | DDC 610.73095496--dc23
LC record available at https://lccn.loc.gov/2019032547
LC ebook record available at https://lccn.loc.gov/2019032548

ISBN 13: 978-1-03-240107-2 (pbk)
ISBN 13: 978-0-367-34425-2 (hbk)
ISBN 13: 978-0-429-32573-1 (ebk)

DOI: 10.4324/9780429325731

Typeset in Times New Roman
by Taylor & Francis Books

Contents

Illustrations

Figures

Tables

Acknowledgements

This book is inspired by the many professional colleagues with whom I have worked and socialised during my professional career in Nepal, the UK and indeed internationally. They currently occupy various positions and fulfil diverse roles, as clinical practitioners, academic researchers, health policy makers and migrant healthcare professionals. In my everyday life, everyone with whom I have interacted has been affected by international nurse migration in one way or another, so it has become everybody's business, and indeed a social norm. This was the wellspring of my research.

First and foremost, I would like to thank all the Nepali nurses, and their families, whom I met in Nepal and in the UK, who shared their deeply personal experiences of being a nurse in Nepal, and in the case of those who have moved to the UK, of their experience of migration. Many granted me their precious time after finishing long shifts, and some after completing night shifts. All nurse *Didi Bahini* and their families have been unfailingly welcoming and extremely accommodating. This book would not have been possible without their unreserved willingness to share their personal experiences with me and, through introducing me to their colleagues, inviting me to join their social world. There are too many to name individually, but I thank them all for their full participation throughout the research process, and continued engagement for many years afterwards, up to the present day.

In Nepal, numerous professional colleagues have been a huge support for me, while I was desperately trying to piece together the complex jigsaw of the politics and new economy around professional nurse education, the capricious labour market and international migration business in the country. Once again there are too many to name; however, I would like to thank senior colleagues, nurse managers in institutions I visited, including the President of the Nursing Association of Nepal and the Board members; staff members at the Centre for Technical Education and Vocational Training, the Nepal Nursing Council, Maharajgunj Nursing Campus, Lalitpur Nursing Campus, Pokhara Nursing Campus, Biratnagar Nursing Campus, and many private colleges, and Thapathali Maternity Hospital, Tribhuwan University Teaching Hospital and many other hospitals. I thank all the nursing students whom I met during my fieldwork. Without their information, it would not have been possible to complete the jigsaw and create a realistic picture of the contemporary situation of professional nursing in Nepal.

I am particularly grateful to Mrs Sabitri Joshi, the late Mrs Lamhoo Amatya and Professor Hari Badan Pradhan, who helped me to dig deeper into some of the previously unexplored parts of the history of nursing in Nepal. I thank Professor Suzanna Mukhia, Professor Sarala Shrestha, Professor Sarala Joshi, Professor Rebecca Sinha, Professor Radha Bangdel, Professor Mana Rai, Professor Chandrakala Sharma and Mrs Rupmati Shrestha, for all their support during my initial fieldwork in Nepal. You not only explained to me the complex politics of the health system but also shared your lunch and drinks with me. I am very grateful to you all.

The Nursing and Midwifery Council (NMC) UK's Public Relations Officer, Ms Polly Kettenacker, provided me with professional records and statistics in 2008–2009, and I wish to thank her for this invaluable information. I also wish to thank Mr Anthony Madu, Customer Information and Data Request Officer at the NMC UK Office for his exceptionally valuable support in unearthing up-to-date data on Nepali nurses' registration status: absolutely key information in this research. Sincere thanks are also due to the Nepalese Nurses Association UK for their great support throughout.

I feel extremely privileged to have been supervised by Professor Kath Melia, and Professor Patricia Jeffery. I am grateful to Professor Ian Harper for all the support I received during my doctoral project. Professor Pam Smith has always been there for me, and I deeply appreciate her encouragement in every aspect in my life. Dr Jeevan Sharma, Mona Adhikari, Linda McKee and Kate Weir have not just been inspiring colleagues, but their longstanding friendship, and continuous prompting, eventually worked and has helped me to complete this book. I have been regularly stimulated and challenged by their very valuable insights into many aspects of international nurse migration and thank them for their in-house intellectual engagement in the subject area. Thank you for being there, particularly during difficult times, and for not letting my motivation falter or run low.

Finally, Tara, my daughter: thank you not only for being patient with me while doing my initial field work, but also for proudly promoting this book and its ideas many months before it finally came into shape. I am also very grateful to my parents, and siblings, and my mother-in-law for encouraging and supporting me wholeheartedly to complete this work.

This book is dedicated to Nepali nurses in particular, but also to all migrant nurses throughout the world.

Abbreviations

ANM	Auxiliary Nurse Midwife
BN	bachelor's degree in nursing
BSc.	bachelor's degree in science
CRB	Criminal Records Bureau
CTEVT	Centre for Technical Education and Vocational Training
DoH	Department of Health (England)
IELTS	International English Language Testing System (a British system)
INGO	International Non-Governmental Organisation
IOM	Institute of Medicine
MN	master's degree in nursing
MoHP	Ministry of Health and Population
NGO	Non-Governmental Organisation
NAN	Nursing Association of Nepal
NNC	Nepal Nursing Council
NMC	Nursing and Midwifery Council (UK)
NVQ	National Vocational Qualification (UK)
ONP	Overseas Nurses Programme
PIN	Professional Identification Number
RCN	Royal College of Nursing (UK)
RGN/RN	Registered General Nurse/Registered Nurse
SLC/SEE	School Leaving Certificate/ Secondary Education Examination
TU	Tribhuwan University
UK	United Kingdom
WHO	World Health Organisation

Introduction

Nursing, gender, and the political economy of female migration in Nepal

In autumn 2008, I met Rita,[1] who worked as a housemaid for an expatriate family in Kathmandu. She had two grown-up daughters and an elderly mother economically dependent upon her. Her elder daughter was at university, studying for an arts degree, while the younger was in her second year of training to be a nurse. When Rita learned that I was a nurse, currently living and working in the UK, and conducting research on Nepali nurses and international migration, she expressed a keen interest in talking to me. For my part, I wanted to talk to her younger daughter; first about why she chose nursing as a career, thereafter about her experiences of being a student nurse, and finally about her future professional aspirations. However, Rita monopolised the conversation, keen to explore the migration possibilities for her daughter, when she finished her training in Nepal. Rita expressed her concerns:

> Gita wanted to do nursing, so first she applied to go to government-run nursing colleges [as they are believed to be better and cheaper]. She applied to Birgunj Nursing Campus. I took her there. I went with her. She then tried to enrol in Bir Hospital Nursing Campus [in Kathmandu]. I supported her with this too. She tried four or five government-funded nursing colleges, but had no luck. She was still determined to join nursing. Finally we had to apply to a private college. She got a place there. She is in the second year of her training now. The fee there is very expensive and it is a big commitment for me. I have to pay a total of 3–4 lakh rupees [approximately £2,500–3,500, based on the current exchange rate at that time]. I work hard to save this amount.

Finally she said her daughter wanted to work as a nurse in Australia, and asked me for advice as to an easier route into international jobs.[2]

International nurse migration in Nepal is an emerging, rapidly growing and highly gendered phenomenon, and has profound implications for gender dynamics within both family and society. International opportunities for professional nurses have become highly desirable, and a 'passport' to a dream job and future life in the affluent West is seen as by far the best career option for a new generation of women in Nepal. In the past 20 years Nepali nurses have become not just more independently mobile, but are now increasingly the 'economic agents', as well as the facilitators, of the international migration of families.

This book is about Nepali nurses, the very first generation of professional women, predominantly from a Hindu society, to have 'dreams' of a professional career, and the possibility thereafter of international migration and the prospect of success and a higher living standard. However, having realised their international migration 'dreams' and aspirations, Nepali nurses have gradually found themselves caught in a set of 'traps' in Britain. UK visa regulations, Nursing and Midwifery Council (NMC) registration and job application processes in the UK have been major barriers to any progress, with an exploitative labour market in the private sector. The resilience of these women, in the face of all their difficulties, has been admirable, with most nurses continuing their struggle to become successful in their personal, social and professional lives in the UK.

For a nurse keen to pursue such dreams, some of the key indicators of success are the securing of an entry visa and a training placement in the UK. The next step is to obtain an NMC UK Professional Identification Number (PIN) or a nursing licence before finally acquiring a post with a work permit. Further dreams are of the opportunity to work in a high-tech modern healthcare system and earn a better salary, thus improving her family's living standard. Achieving higher education and creating future career opportunities for her children and other family members are further goals. However, those with such dreams encounter difficulties at every step of their career trajectory. After illustrating the pitfalls in their actual migration process, this book demonstrates how nurses navigate their way out of each of the 'traps' in the UK's healthcare labour market, as they journey towards attaining their goals. It also chronicles how they adapt to new social and professional environments and make new lives here.

Nursing, gender and the political economy of female migration in Nepal

Nursing has become one of the most attractive and highly competitive female professions in Nepal today. Professional education is in high demand, and indeed nursing has been perceived as both a respectable and an ideal career for many educated young women, predominantly those from middle-class backgrounds. This is because, in recent decades, this profession has facilitated Nepali nurses' entry into the global healthcare labour market: a dream job, not only for young nurses, but also for their families.

Since 2000, there has been a phenomenal growth in the country's training capacity to cater for the growing number of applicants in nurse education. Nurse production has been so high that the country's health system has not been able to absorb all of the new graduates. After completing their professional education and obtaining their licence from the Nepal Nursing Council

(NNC), some nurses contribute to Nepal's healthcare sector. However, in the past two decades increasing numbers of Nepali nurses have also crossed national borders to participate in the global healthcare labour market. Those with sufficient family support to finance their nursing education abroad travel to India, and in increasing numbers, to Australia. On obtaining professional qualifications from foreign universities, they seek job opportunities in the wider healthcare market internationally.

The international nurse migration literature suggests that most conventional migrations have historical links, with socio-cultural and language factors stimulating human mobility and facilitating relocation (Castle 2000; Massey et al. 2006; Choy 2003). For Nepali nurses there are no historical or colonial links with the countries that are currently the preferred destinations: Australia, New Zealand, the UK and the USA. Nepal has a long tradition of international migration, with Nepali men being leaders in migration and small numbers of dependent women and children following them (Seddon et al. 2001). The new trend of international nurse migration has also reversed this phenomenon: now nurses take the lead followed by their husbands, children and other close relatives (Adhikari 2013).

As Gita's story above illustrates, in Nepal international nurse migration is a family affair. Nurses require a great deal of family support and guidance to make decisions and they continue to need support when relocating and settling in their chosen destination country. To begin with, family support is needed to finance girls' secondary education and then their nursing education, even before they can plan an international move. Family support is required at every stage of the nurse migration journey: from choosing a destination country, preparing for travel and paying for relocation costs in the destination country, and providing continued support and maintenance thereafter. The support nurses need is not only monetary but is also emotional. It includes taking responsibility for the care of those dependent family members left behind, be they young children or elderly parents.

At the same time, the practicalities of migrating internationally are complex. It requires detailed knowledge of the opportunities available abroad. Most importantly, aspiring nurses need to know how to overcome the destination country-specific bureaucratic and regulatory challenges. To meet this demand there is now a thriving new market of International Education Consultancies (IECs). Many nurses turn to these 'agents' or brokers to manage all the practicalities. IECs facilitate Nepali nurses' departure abroad and help them to prepare official documents needed for migration, such as course or job acceptance letters from a foreign university or employer, and also assist in the preparation of bank statements. Among the services they offer are visa and interview preparation training and English language courses. They also compile Chartered Accountant (CA) and police reports. In short, they manage all the practical issues, subject to an exorbitant service charge. As such there is an emerging new economy around professional nursing and international nurse migration, both in Nepal and globally (Adhikari 2010; Kingma 2006).

Key arguments

This book presents four inter-linking arguments that explain the current international nurse migration phenomenon in Nepal. These emerge empirically from the participants' real-life experiences of having been nurses in Nepal and the overall experience of their migration journeys, and thereafter from being at the margin of the UK's health system, as well as from available literature in the field of international nurse migration. These are: (1) professional nursing has been a catalyst for changing social and gender dynamics in Nepal, (2) the global nursing shortage and international migration are gender issues, (3) privatisation in healthcare systems makes for labour market vulnerability and stimulates international recruitment of health professionals, and (4) international nurse migration is part of the process of globalisation in health.

Professional nursing and changing social and gender dynamics in Nepal

Nursing began to be a very attractive female profession in Nepal in the 1990s, at a time of profound socio-political change took place in the country, including changes in gender politics. Coinciding with the major political shift, from a party-less *Panchayat* system to multi-party democracy, debates around women's rights, women's health and female literacy became, and remain, political and development priorities (Ahern 2004). Women's newfound mobility, both nationally and internationally, has gradually become a social norm (Adhikari 2013; Adhikari & Melia 2013; Brusle 2010). Since then, increasing numbers of women are moving away from home for education or work (SWiFT 2017; Hamal-Gurung 2015; Adhikari 2010; UNIFEM & NIDS 2006). As a female-only profession (as of the 2018–2019 academic year), nursing offers an excellent example of how women's social position is changing, and how increasingly they are becoming their families' breadwinners and the lead actors in family migration.

Despite the fact that the total number of nurses licensed to practise in Nepal is comparatively small, being to date only 82,388[3] (NNC 2019), they are highly sought after socially, as desirable marriage partners for young educated Nepali men from middle-class families. The traditional arranged marriage system is gradually changing, and now nurses can have a say when it comes to making marriage decisions. Families now seek suitable nurse brides for their sons: a major shift in gender relations in Nepali society.

Only one generation ago, *Chhori Bigrye Nurse-le, Chhora Bigrye Commerce-le* [daughters are corrupted by being nurses and sons by studying commerce] was a common saying in Nepal. Nursing was then a relatively new profession for the vast majority of people and had yet to gain social recognition, acceptance and respect. Although nurses at that time were from relatively educated and, in the majority, from high caste families, the saying was a common one across many classes and in many social groups. Because of the nature of nursing, which involved staying away from the family and regularly working at night, it was not deemed the most desirable of jobs. It was also not considered socially acceptable for a young woman to move away from home, as this could potentially ruin the family *Ijjet*, or honour (Maxwell with Sinha 2004).

By the beginning of the twenty-first century negative attitudes towards nursing had completely changed. Now with widening access to the profession for women from diverse castes and socio-economic backgrounds, a nursing qualification is not only seen as a possible guarantee of a job in Nepal, but is also viewed as a licence to work abroad in affluent countries (Baral & Sapkota 2015; Thapa 2009). Nurses are becoming independent, mobile and enjoying more freedom. They have considerably more bargaining power within their households. Nevertheless, despite this significant level of independence, both financially as well as in taking part in major life decisions for themselves, their life trajectories are still heavily influenced by their family's aspirations. As already noted, international nurse migration in Nepal remains a major family affair and professional nursing has been a catalyst for a change in gender relations and socio-economic mobility, across existing castes and social classes in Nepal.

Global nursing shortages and international nurse migration are gender issues

Feminist scholars argue that 'care work', both paid and unpaid, is socially sanctioned work for women, both traditionally and also in modern times. Nursing is a caring profession and has always been included in this care work category, as the major aspect of nursing involves looking after and caring for children, for ill or frail people and for the elderly and the disabled in society (Zimmerman et al. 2006; Kingma 2006; Spitzer et al. 2006). It has been a female-dominated profession globally, and a 'female-only' profession in Nepal.

With the socio-political changes that emerged after the Second World War, women in many affluent countries obtained better-paid work, as well as a wider choice of job opportunities in society. As a consequence the attraction towards domestic work and care work, including nursing, has declined generally, creating a care vacuum, particularly at the most basic level of looking after young children and the elderly. From the 1970s, as Ehrenreich & Russell-Hochschild (2002) argue, increasing numbers of women from developing countries have been employed to take up domestic and care work posts in affluent countries. They come to look after other people's children, and the sick and elderly, whilst leaving their own young children, sick and elderly behind. This type of female migration from resource-poor countries to provide care to people in the affluent countries has been described as a 'care drain' (Zimmerman et al. 2006; Ehrenreich & Russell-Hochschild 2002). This global 'care drain' has of course created a need for a 'care chain' to support those who are left behind (Sassen 2006).

Nursing and care work is physically and emotionally demanding, involves unsocial working hours and is generally poorly paid. Kingma (2006) highlights that the profession is dominated by females, and is less well-paid than male-dominated or mixed-gender professions. Due to this and because, at its heart, it is care work, nursing has been neglected and remains a low-paid profession globally. While the attraction towards nursing and care work in affluent countries is declining, the need for it is increasing because of demographic changes. There are increasing numbers of elderly people, combined with rising healthcare expectations and needs (Cangiano et al. 2009). Ageing populations, declining birth rates and shrinking workforce pools, combined with a lack of workforce planning and inadequate financing in healthcare systems, are the main reasons for global nursing shortages. These shortages have stimulated nurse migration from low-income countries to affluent ones (WHO 2006).

Privatisation and commoditisation of the health service and its labour market vulnerability

Globally, healthcare has increasingly been privatised and commoditised. Since the late 1980s, as part of governments' strategies to restructure health services to deal with budget deficits, the private sector has been invited into health service provision in the UK, Nepal and most countries in the world (Pollock 2005). Privatisation in nurse education in Nepal and the recruitment of nurses and health professionals from the global labour market by the UK illustrate this phenomenon (Adhikari 2011; Pollock 2005; Buchan 2000). As a result of poor workforce planning by the government(s) and gradual privatisation, the global healthcare labour market has become highly volatile. This book focuses on Nepali nurses' real life experiences, both at home in Nepal, as well as in the UK's healthcare labour market.

There is an urgent need for more nurses and care workers globally. Rather than timely and effective workforce planning, improving working terms and conditions, making nursing an attractive profession and improving retention locally and nationally, affluent countries have been recruiting nurses from resource-poor countries. Migrant nurses and care workers have been used as a cheap workforce to fill hard-to-fill care work posts. Affluent countries have been criticised for 'commoditising' nursing in this manner, and not investing in their own provision of an urgently needed workforce. Using cheap labour, from economically disadvantaged countries, renders care work a commodity that can be bought and sold in the contemporary global healthcare market (Kingma 2006; Zimmerman et al. 2006; Herdman 2004; Stillwell et al. 2004).

Care and the assistance of a care worker are readily available nowadays, for those who can afford to pay. This challenges the fundamental principle of health care as a right for all individuals, not just for those who can buy it. Critics view this trend as 'picking staff off the shelves', for employing healthcare professionals has come to resemble supermarket shopping (Smith & Mackintosh 2007).

The British economy has been the main driver of its healthcare labour market, and dictates its immigration policy. Healthcare professionals are recruited and the immigration policy is relaxed, or tightened as it suits the country at the time. The UK has failed to show any consideration of the potential impact on the low-income source countries from which it is recruiting health professionals. Other international nurse recruiting nations, such as the USA and Australia, have failed too and these issues have aroused much global ethical and political debate. These factors contribute to fluctuations in the healthcare labour market. This book documents Nepali nurses' precarious migration journeys from one volatile labour market in Nepal to yet another in the UK, a volatility which impacts greatly on how well they are accepted and integrated, both socially and professionally.

Nurse and health professional migration as a part of globalisation in health

Globalisation scholars argue that the world is becoming increasingly inter-connected. Modern communication systems allow news, messages and events in one part of the world to be instantly transmitted across vast distances. Healthcare products and drugs are produced in one corner of the world to be used somewhere else, often thousands of miles away. Disease-causing organisms have no barriers; they can cross national borders quickly. SARS, Multi Drug Resistant (MDR) TB, and Swine Flu (H1N1 virus) are examples of this. Nursing and healthcare jobs are advertised online and suitable candidates are recruited from the wider global labour market. Health services themselves in some countries are tailored for global consumers. Medical tourism in Thailand and Cuba, telemedicine facilities in private hospitals in Kathmandu, increasing numbers of multinational companies providing private health services such as eye care and care of the elderly services in Britain (Tschudin & Davis 2008; Pollock 2005; Buse et al. 2005), are just a few examples of how globally interdependent we are, and of the globalisation in health in the twenty-first century.

There are many interlinking facets. Economic, cultural, media and techno-logical globalisation all directly affect healthcare systems and have no national boundaries. Money is invested and trade agreements are made at global, as well as increasingly at regional levels. Some of these trade agreements on goods and services facilitate regional movements of people. For example, freedom to move and work within the countries in the European Union (EU) and the Caribbean Communities (CARICOM) is made possible by such agreements (Kingma 2006). The migration of health professionals is a part of this whole process. Currently China, India, Indonesia and Nepal are trying to produce thousands of surplus nurses for international supply (Adhikari 2014; Matsuno 2008; Khadria 2007). Indeed China, India and the Philippines have entered into a bilateral agreement with the UK government in the international recruitment of health professionals for the UK (Buchan et al. 2009). Japan has made bilateral economic partnership agreements with Indonesia, Vietnam and the Philippines and recruited nurses from there to fill nursing vacancies (Carlos 2012; Matsuno 2008; Connell 2008). Nurses are not only moving from south to north globally, but new regional patterns are emerging too. There is no country whose health system is not affected by global events and policies. One can see globalisation in health everywhere, be it in the movement of peoples, in scientific inventions, in distance or online learning, and of course in the migration of health professionals. The migration of Nepali nurses to the UK, USA and Australia is just part of this kaleidoscopic pattern – of globalisation in health.

Origin of this study in my own research journey

In August 2000 I returned to the UK from a two-year stay in my home country of Nepal, to live in Oxford with my family. After settling there, I started to look for a part-time nursing post. Initially, I was quite apprehensive about going back to work for a number of reasons. Principally, I would have to leave our two-year-old daughter behind, and this was never going to be easy. Additionally, I felt my professional nursing skills were becoming 'rusty' and that I needed to re-orientate myself to recent changes within the profession. I joined a nursing agency and in fact found my return to clinical practice easier than I had expected. Within a few weeks however I began to note the many interesting changes in the local nursing workforce situation.

Working with the agency in different healthcare facilities, I met many internationally educated nurses. At the time, local and national shortages of nurses in hospitals was a hot topic, alongside lengthening hospital waiting lists and the consequent increased recruitment of nurses from international sources. Oxford's John Radcliffe NHS Trust had recently recruited many Filipino nurses. I worked with some of them, along with many others from a wide range of countries: Kenya, Australia, South Africa, India and Zimbabwe. There were regular reports in the British media on changes within the NHS, and close coverage of Tony Blair's promise to recruit 20,000 more nurses by 2004, in order to reduce hospital waiting lists. As a result, by 2001–2002, there were more internationally educated nurses registered with the Nursing Midwifery Council (NMC) UK than home-trained nurses. From the position of being an insider within the professional environment, I heard many interesting stories and listened to a great deal of gossip, as a part of occupational socialising. Some accounts were positive and others negative. I learned particularly that some internationally recruited nurses were being exploited in private nursing homes. One particular encounter with a nurse drew my attention and affected me greatly for several years afterwards.

One spring day in 2001, the nursing agency phoned me and asked me if I could work a shift at a particular nursing home in Oxford city. They added that this home always had plenty of work available; and that, if I wanted, I could work there for as many hours as I liked. I accepted this assignment, keen to see what it would be like to work there. On joining the staff the next day for the morning shift, I soon realised that some staff had permanent contracts, whilst others were agency staff, there just for a day like myself. We received the night report and started our day shift.

There was one other nurse working with me that day: Mary, a qualified nurse from Hungary who had been working there for some time. I was told that Mary knew the place well so she would be able to support me when I needed anything. Within a few hours of working with her, I learned a great deal about her situation and the home's staff recruitment practice. She had been working as a carer there, a job below her professional expertise (she indicated), because she did not have NMC-UK registration. She had been recruited directly from Hungary, along with a team of staff from various categories, from carers to kitchen staff, drivers and cleaners, to work in a number of nursing homes in Oxfordshire, privately owned and managed by the same private company. Some other staff members informed me that the owner and the manager of this nursing home business went to Hungary on a regular basis to recruit nurses and other support staff directly from there. Once in the UK, staff were given fixed-term contracts, usually for one or two years. Accommodation was provided by the management, but at a cost. When a new batch of staff arrived in Heathrow, the manager would arrange for them to be picked up from the airport and taken to their pre-arranged accommodation.

Mary and some of the other carers I worked with that morning were, as noted above, part of a larger group of staff, of various categories, recruited to work in this nursing home. Mary had a two-year contract to work there and, when I met her, she had been there for almost 18 months. Part of her contract was that she would receive initially an in-house adaptation course,[4] and then she could register with the NMC-UK.[5] She would be able thereafter to obtain a staff nurse position in this nursing home. But time passed and this did not happen, she told me. This was because there was no mentor available to support her with the process. She was disappointed and very unhappy working there. She felt exploited working a 12-hour day, for five or six days a week, on a low wage, but said she was unable to change her job. When I asked why she could not just leave this place, she told me her passport had been taken away and was being kept by the management. The informal practice of this management was to keep foreign employees' passports until the end of their contract period, and Mary still had six more months to wait, and to endure. I felt very strongly that the management's actions were morally wrong. I felt angry and helpless, as I could do nothing about it, as although many staff members were miserable about their working conditions, they were not supposed to discuss them with outsiders. They were scared of being deported back home. Working there was a very unpleasant experience, and after a week I decided I could not accept further assignment there and continue to feel so angry and sad. I stayed in touch with some of the staff, however, and over the next year heard further dismaying and horrifying stories of their unacceptably poor working conditions.

The following year I went to Nepal for a short family visit. On meeting some of my friends and former work colleagues I realised there had also been a major change within the country's nursing profession. I was approached by some senior nurses, some of whom wanted to come to the UK, as they had heard that there were many nursing opportunities available here. Others were exploring possible business opportunities and setting up networks to facilitate nurse migration. Their idea was that they would set up a recruiting agency in Nepal, with the purpose of sending nurses to the UK. They further proposed that I, at the UK end, would link up with them to find jobs for Nepali nurses. I learned that networks like this were already established and fully functioning in Kathmandu, but that they were not able to deal with the increasing volume of nurse candidates interested in trying to move to the UK.

I began to realise the magnitude of professional and social changes that had happened within a short period in Nepal. Looking back to just about two and a half decades ago, when I entered the nursing profession in the early 1980s, my grandfather was totally against the idea of me (a teenage girl) leaving home and moving to Kathmandu, to live in a completely strange place with strangers, without any guardian there. He feared that I might find a boy from a different caste and run away with him, or write love letters to a man. There would be no family member to control and safeguard my behaviour. Preserving family honour, caste and cultural values was desirable behaviour for all, but 'a must' for a young unmarried girl. So, to my grandfather, the idea of my training as a nurse seemed totally inappropriate and presented a risk of ruining his family reputation. This was not just a worry for my grandfather and some of my relatives but for many other families in the 1980s, even though nursing was a female only profession.[6] All student nurses were given female only accommodation, with a female warden in place 24/7 to safeguard and oversee trainee nurses' behaviour. We had no choice but to stay there during our three-year training period. Visitors were not allowed on the premises, and we were only allowed to go out from 10 a.m. until 4 p.m. once a week on Saturdays, if granted special permission from the 'house-mother', the hostel warden. At the time there were two staff nurse colleges in the country, educating only 50 nurses a year.

Professional nursing started to change from the late 1980s. The major political shift of 1990 and the establishment of multi-party democracy in the country led to the new democratic government encouraging private sector involvement in education, health, and many other development activities. Since then, the social perception of, and the attraction towards, nursing has changed. Given greater publicity for the education sector in general, as well as for nurse education, there was an exponential increase in demand for nurse training courses. Accommodation rules have become much more relaxed and it is not compulsory for student nurses to be in female-only accommodation. Today they can choose where to live during their training: in their own homes with their families or in rented flats in town. From that time young, educated usually urban girls seemed to gain more freedom and parents and grandparents became less concerned about them becoming nurses and leaving home. Parents and grandparents now in fact support and encourage nurses to seek international opportunities.

Due to the increased demand for nurse education places, many new programmes have been set up within the last decade. Indeed many of my friends and colleagues seemed very busy with new job opportunities in these new colleges. Having observed all these changes and learned of Nepali nurses' dreams of migrating to the UK, the idea of this research began to form. I was also witness to some of the working realities in the UK, and had continued to notice further changes in its healthcare system as regards nursing and the workforce situation. Over the next few years I saw increasing numbers of Nepali nurses coming to the UK, and was particularly struck by the fact that many highly educated nurses, with master's level education and many years of managerial and clinical experience in Nepal, came to the UK to find no corresponding jobs were available, and that they were prepared to work at a much lower grade than they had done back home.

This book, then, is the result of my doctoral ethnography (2005–2010) and personal and professional experience of nursing in Nepal and the UK. It is based on my research into Nepali nurses' experiences of migration to the UK, and my continued engagement in this field up to the present day. I address two broad questions, the first of which asks 'how and why do Nepali nurses migrate to the UK?' The second question is 'how do they materialise and experience the whole migration process: professionally and personally and also socially?' For migration involves acceptance of and adaptation to a new working environment forbye the negotiation of all the related hurdles. Nurses have to lead their family's migration as well as cope with resentment on several fronts.

Research approach and practicalities

I began the study by following nurses' professional journeys from Nepal to the UK, not in the sense that I physically travelled with them, but I collected their current and retrospective migration experiences. I visited nursing education institutions in Nepal relevant to nurses' professional lives. In order to further understand the professional context in Nepal, I traced the history of nursing there and mapped out major changes in the profession. The starting point of my study of participants' journeys has been their entry into professional education and their educational background in general. Their destination, and the end point of this particular research, is the UK, where Nepali nurses have been living and working since their arrival here: Nepali nurses' migration is contextualised as a part of larger global changes in healthcare systems. It is part of the globalisation and the systematic and gradual privatisation in healthcare labour market conditions and its relation to international nurse migration.

Since my engagement with this research in 2005, I have met with my research participants, in both Nepal and the UK and, as above noted, visited many relevant institutions in their everyday or 'natural settings' (Ritchie & Lewis 2003; Brewer 2000; Gellner & Hirsch 2001; Handwerker 2001). I personally gathered all the research information, using multiple research techniques including observation, in-depth interviews, and focus group discussions with wider groups of participants. In addition, I had numerous formal and informal discussions with participants, and reviewed all available relevant records and policy documents. Initial fieldwork was conducted between the summer of 2006 and December 2009, with a subsequent number, to date, of many years of continued engagement with professional colleagues in Nepal and with migrant nurse colleagues in the UK.

In Nepal

Initial fieldwork for my doctoral study in Nepal was conducted in three stages and followed-up in three visits (in 2010, 2012 and 2013) with further regular updating of the situation until spring 2019. From August to December 2006, I mapped out the nursing colleges and universities in Nepal, visited some of them, and met with key stakeholders in the nursing sector. I visited the Nursing Association of Nepal (NAN), the Nepal Nursing Council (NNC), and the Centre for Technical Education and Vocational Training (CTEVT), the Ministry of Health and Population (MoHP) of Nepal and numerous nursing colleges. There I met student nurses, qualified nurses, academics, senior nurses working at policy level, and nurse political activists. I also had some email communication with British Embassy staff in the visa section in Kathmandu. At that time British visa processing had yet to be outsourced to a private company (VSF Global). Additionally, I visited some high profile IECs or agencies specialising in brokering nurses abroad.

During my doctoral fieldwork I visited a total of 20 nursing colleges in Nepal. Four of them had kept a register and recorded whether their former graduates had gone abroad, or initiated the migration process, but only if a foreign nursing authority had requested verification of their nursing qualification. On review the majority of requests were from the licensing authorities of many American States; from the NMC-UK; and from the nursing councils of Australia, New Zealand, and Canada. I met senior academic faculty members for informal discussions, and also met with B.Sc. nursing students in their classroom for a group discussion about why they had chosen to study nursing and their future aspirations.

I travelled to Nepal for further fieldwork in July and August 2007 and resumed my research there in October, through November and December of that year. At that time I visited nursing colleges I had not visited before and revisited others for updates on progress and changes within the institutions. Additionally, I visited Pokhara, a town in west-central Nepal, where there are three nursing programmes, and was able to gather research data from one. I went to east Nepal, to the industrial town of Biratnagar and to Dharan. Of the six programmes in this region I visited four. A further visit was to the

CTEVT, where I met officers from the Exam Division, the Training Accreditation Division, and the Research and Information Division respectively. The final update visit was conducted between August and December 2009. I again revisited some of the colleges for updates, as well as some new colleges not previously researched. I was invited to a meeting organised by NAN, and this and other social events in which I participated were equally valuable as regards giving me further insight into the issues involved in international nurse migration.

Subsequent follow-up visits were made in 2010, 2012, 2013 and then annually for the next four years (2014–2019). During these visits I gathered new data on changes in nursing education and the labour market situation in Nepal. I have regularly reviewed available college records of nurses in the process of migration, in order to capture changing patterns, in terms of numbers involved and the destinations of migrating Nepali nurses. I also have been involved in teaching qualitative research methods in two nursing colleges in the Kathmandu valley as a guest lecturer, the most recent session being in 2018. I have continued to engage with the study of professional nursing education in Nepal and am aware of policy and the practice environment there.

Research in the UK

During my doctoral fieldwork in the UK, I met over 100 Nepali migrant nurses during the three-year study period (2006–2009), employing a 'snowballing' technique (Ritchie & Lewis 2003). I formally interviewed 22 nurses, as my main informants. In addition, I have had numerous informal discussions, countless telephone conversations and multiple meetings with a number of informants. I have remained in touch from 2007 to date with many of my informants, and also with the Nepalese Nurse Association UK, a diaspora organisation which was set up by some of the informants of my initial study.

Twenty-one interviews were recorded with permission from the participants. One nurse was happy to be interviewed but was very shy and therefore declined to be tape-recorded. There were three instances when nurses asked me to turn the recorder off before sharing personal and sensitive information with me. I spent between four and six hours, sometimes longer, with each nurse I interviewed, using an open-ended and simple interview guide. Observational methods and informal discussions helped me gain a deeper insight into nurses' professional and social lives in the UK. In addition I met with a nursing home manager in England, who had provided adaptation training placements for 78 Nepali nurses, and an NHS nurse manager in Scotland. She used to be responsible for recruiting and training internationally educated nurses, as part of the 2000–2004 international recruitment drive, before the NMC introduced the Overseas Nurses Programme in 2006.

The purpose of the research interviews was explained to all participants. They were all fully informed and aware that they could withdraw from the research at any time if they felt uncomfortable. Apart from some key public figures, most of the participants I interviewed in the UK have been anonymised to protect their identities.

I visited nurses in Oxford and nearby villages; Riding Mill in Northumberland; London; Watford; East Sussex; and Swansea. In Scotland I met with nurses in Central Scotland and in Aberdeen and Edinburgh. Interviews were conducted in a mixture of both Nepali and English. More than half of the conversations in the UK were in English, as many informants felt comfortable using English words and often whole sentences. In Nepal, too, many English words are adopted and widely used by qualified nurses. Some senior managers were fluent in English. I later, however, transcribed and translated the Nepali recordings into English.

Insider/outsider context of this research

Traditionally in an ethnographic study, researchers from 'outside' would come to study people in their 'natural' settings. However, it is increasingly common to study one's own world and in different organisational settings (Gellner & Hirsch 2001). In this study, I, as a Nepali nurse, currently working and living in Britain, studied Nepali nurses' migration to the UK. I see myself as a 'participant insider' as I also socialise with Nepali migrant nurses in the UK (Mosse 2005). As Mosse argues, 'the social processes of an organisation are better understood from within' (2005: 11).

Being an insider has raised a number of issues, not least the position it places me in relation to my research participants. I share the experiences of my research participants: the overall experience of being trained in Nepal and becoming a migrant nurse in British healthcare settings. This has undoubtedly been a huge asset. I felt privileged that the nurses I met were happy to talk to me, and I had easy access to them. I also had unprecedented access to nursing colleges and other relevant institutions in Nepal, because of friends and colleagues from my previous posts who now occupy senior positions in various institutions. This 'old friends' network' has certainly facilitated my access to an inside knowledge of the organisations I studied.

I have been working in the UK healthcare system since 1994, and I have a good understanding of professional nursing registration regulations and processes and, most importantly, recent changes within the healthcare system. Generally, ethnographers spend a long time learning the language and culture of their study population (Gellner & Hirsch 2001). My main advantage is that I speak, read and write Nepali and English fluently, and this has been invaluable. Language and cultural difficulties were minimal on both sides, in comparison to what they would have been, if I had been an outsider conducting this study.

The whole process of researching this book has not been totally smooth nor without difficulties. Nepal has been undergoing a series of major political crises since the start of the Maoist War in 1996, and remains unsettled until now, at the time of writing. Since 1996 indeed, the country has had two states of emergency declared by the former king, and numerous changes of government. I found doing fieldwork, particularly at turbulent times in the earlier stage of my research, all very slow and frustrating. I had just arrived in Nepal in 2006 to begin my fieldwork when there was a government change, just after the country was declared a republic. The Health Minister was removed from his position with the change of the entire parliament, and many key positions within the nursing sector filled by ministry-level nominations became vacant. At the same time the President, Vice-President and all NNC board members were removed from their positions. When I visited the NNC in August 2006, there had been no NNC board member for almost four months, except for that of the Registrar. Her contract was terminated with the others, but she was appointed again very quickly for urgent work only. Only a few administrative staff remained, as their posts were not affected. The Registrar was mostly occupied with professional registration and administration, but all professional regulation and strengthening work was on hold. This affected my work too.

To make matters worse, in 2006, during the first phase of my research fieldwork, there was a long-term strike by CTEVT students, which involved many private nursing colleges. The CTEVT office was closed, and in fact the dispute also led to a general strike by CTEVT staff. The council chairman had been removed with the old government. The staff union had disapproved the interim appointment of a chairman, so his office was padlocked and staff were all on strike. This lasted for months and affected my visits to various key institutions. There had also been frequent, unplanned street protests, blockades, and demonstrations by students and the youth forces of various political parties, amongst others. Although I did not personally feel particularly unsafe during my fieldwork in Nepal, the frequent interruptions meant I had to take any opportunities available while gathering research information, as and when possible. In recent years the political situation has improved slowly, with fewer street protests and less unrest.

In Nepal it is almost impossible to plan and arrange times to meet people. It has become a recognised aspect of the nation's working culture. Consequently, in order to meet and interview key stakeholders I have had to be extremely flexible, and always ready to respond when the opportunity does present itself.

In the UK, although difficulties with timings were fairly minor, they did exist, and I had to adjust to them and always remain flexible. I travelled long distances to meet Nepali nurses who worked long days and shifts with unsocial hours. Many of the nurses I met had little free time and I had to fit around their working hours. Although the majority of nurses were always very willing to be interviewed and very accommodating, it has been difficult to use their only day off in a week for this research. For example, some nurses I interviewed in the UK worked five or six nights a week, with just one or two nights off. After finishing night shift they would need to sleep during the day, so arranging to meet them posed a challenge. For example, I was in East Sussex twice for initial fieldwork, the first time for two days and the second time for four days, and all the time I was there, some nurses I had intended to see were working night shifts or working longer days (12-hour shifts), and I was not able to meet them. They were genuinely very busy and tired. My long-term engagement with Nepali nurses here has facilitated a full appreciation of how they live their new lives and have settled in the UK.

Emotional and ethical challenges

Quite often I have been in emotionally uncomfortable situations. I felt that I have been seen as a contact point for aspiring Nepali nurses; an *Afno-man-chhe* (of one's own people) and this has raised some expectations, quite understandably perhaps. *Afno-manchhe* networks are vital in Nepali society and usually work quite well too. During the fieldwork for this research, both in Nepal and the UK, I was, and still am, regularly approached by nurses who desperately want to migrate, to work in the UK, Australia, New Zealand or the US. Unfortunately, I have never been in a position to facilitate their migration. I am asked for guidance as to how they might achieve their ambitions, but again have not been in a position to advise them. I try to explain UK working regulations, only to learn this is not what they seek. I often feel useless in terms of my inability to meet their needs and help them. Given my knowledge of overseas nurses' working conditions in the UK, I would like to have advised them not to come. However, I could see how keen the nurses were, and was reluctant therefore to discourage their dreams of an international career. I felt that the whole migration process might mean years of being on an emotional rollercoaster, as well as living in 'two worlds' (Philogene 2008). This issue is explored further.

During the initial research field work in the UK, some Nepali nurses contacted me to help them find adaptation training placements and jobs, as their visas were about to expire and, if they failed to find a placement soon, they would need to go back home, but I was unable to help them. In the UK, there were genuinely not enough training placements available for internationally educated nurses. I felt quite helpless yet again, given the difficult and stressful circumstances in which they found themselves.

Another important factor was that the nature of nursing work undertaken in the UK could be a possible source of embarrassment. Some of the Nepali nurses I met were very experienced and had held senior and permanent government positions at home. However, in the UK they were working as night nurses in the least desirable nursing sectors, such as care of the elderly or in psychiatric institutions, or were doing work far below the level of their clinical skills, experience and professional education. These were sensitive issues that would perhaps have been easier for an 'outsider' researcher to explore and discuss more openly. Finally, some nurses were on student visas, and were unsure as to whether their visas would allow them to engage in full-time work. Due to this issue being so sensitive, some appeared reluctant to meet with me and discuss their experiences in detail.

The majority of managers of nursing education institutions in Nepal have affiliations with major political parties. Social and political networks are very important in Nepal and nursing society is still relatively small and close. Senior nurses, educated some time ago, are easily identifiable and so would not remain anonymous. Being a part of this network has facilitated some openings and closed others, while an outside researcher would have had a quite different experience. I believe that coming from a high caste Brahmin family is less relevant in this regard, as my participants are professionals from the new middle-class society (Liechty 2003) and caste is not as important an issue for my research as local politics.

Chapter outlines

Chapter 1 provides a detailed context of nurse education and the healthcare labour market situation, mainly since the establishment of the profession in the mid-1950s until the present day in Nepal. As highlighted above, international opportunities for professional nurses are regarded as the most desirable, and nursing qualifications are seen as 'passports to a foreign job'. Young Nepali nurses are not just becoming increasingly mobile nationally and internationally, but also are becoming 'economic agents', as well as facilitators, for the international migration of their families. It has become common knowledge too that many successful, young and educated men now look for nurse-brides. As a result of women's changing position in society and a phenomenal change in social perceptions of nursing, the demand for nurse education places is growing.

To meet this increased demand, there has been a rapid growth in Nepal's nursing education capacity since the 1990s. The private sector has been a key player in providing nurse education and has grown beyond belief, and the state has not been able to effectively regulate this growth. The discussion in this chapter raises a major question about the quality of nurse education in the private sector, particularly in a resource-constrained environment. Nursing education and healthcare has been seen as a profit making industry. The reality is that more nurses are educated every year and more nurses are leaving Nepal for international jobs, thus illustrating how the global labour demand impacts on nurse education, the labour market situation and ultimately healthcare provision in Nepal today.

Chapter 2 explores the issue of nurse migration decision-making, planning and preparation for migration. The main focus is on women's agency in migration decision-making processes, in addition to the political economy of international nurse migration. The chapter begins by illustrating how professional women are able to make migration decisions, albeit with the 'influence' and support of their families and friends. A detailed discussion ensues on how International Educational Consultancies (IECs) or migration brokers facilitate nurses' moves, and navigate bureaucratic hurdles related to visa and work permit regulations in the UK. The various steps of obtaining nursing qualifications in Nepal, then the necessary visas and work permits, and finally a nursing licence to work in the UK, are all complex processes. Nurses often take short-cut routes, as guided by IEC agents, friends and colleagues and other informal social networks. Quite often, their migration dreams are so powerful that they choose the most likely route for obtaining any kind of entry visa to the UK.

From Chapter 3, the book focuses on Nepali nurses' lives in the UK, from the time of their arrival. It explores where they first go on arrival, their initial experiences of settling in, and how they source any existing support networks in the UK. How Nepal-educated nurses fit into the British healthcare system is discussed, for there are different regulations for nurses educated within EU countries and those from Commonwealth countries. This situation of course may change after brexit negotiations are fully implemented. Nursing jobs in the UK are first for UK-educated, then EU-educated nurses, and after this for those outside the EU. There is no mechanism guaranteeing a job and an appropriate work permit for Nepali nurses. Their real life case stories, as presented here, illustrate their challenging journeys towards obtaining nursing posts and work permits, regularly perceived by nurses as 'traps'.

The discussion in this chapter suggests that Nepali nurses are perhaps more vulnerable to exploitation in the private sector, as the door to the NHS is closed. This is because of the Department of Health in England's 'Code of Practice for the International Recruitment of Healthcare Professionals' (DoH 2004), which placed Nepal on the list of banned countries, from which recruitment of health workers has been considered unethical. Nepal is not a Commonwealth country and Nepali nurses seem to be getting a 'bad deal' in the UK's nursing labour market. For some Nepali nurses, overcoming the hurdles of gaining a UK nursing licence (an NMC-PIN), finding a job and securing a work permit has seemed like *Kahilei Nasakkine Samasyaharuko Sikri* – 'a never-ending chain of difficulties'. Nevertheless, nurses remain determined to overcome these challenges, to try to realise their 'dreams'.

Chapter 4 further examines Nepali nurses and their professional lives and professional assimilation in the UK: their expectations and the reality. Nurses explain their working relationships with colleagues, patients and with their line-managers. Many Nepali nurses have been disappointed with the working conditions and types of work they have found in the UK, particularly in the private care home sector. Almost all of the study participants had initially experienced downward professional mobility. Many were highly qualified and had many years of management experience, some with very specialist clinical skills, yet have ended up doing very basic, non-nursing types of work, experiencing another set of 'traps'. Their dreams and expectations of working in a medically and technologically advanced healthcare system have failed totally. Their qualifications, skills and experiences have been misplaced in the UK working environment, particularly in the private sector. Increasingly they are led to feel they have been deskilled and are now members of a marginal workforce in the UK health system.

In Chapter 5 migrant nurses express their disappointment in their lives in the Diaspora. It details their experience of further 'traps' and how they have navigated a way out of them towards more positive experiences and some hopes for the future. The chapter highlights the numerous hidden costs during the early period of migration, such as the pain of family separation and the barriers that hinder family reunion. Even after reunion, new family challenges emerge. Nurses' husbands are not used to being socially and economically dependent on their wives in Nepal, but must adjust to their changing social status and lives as dependent husbands in the UK. To add insult to injury, many of them have had no choice but to accept unskilled jobs in the UK, after giving up highly respectable positions in Nepal. For some dependent husbands migration brings only downward social mobility, frustration, disappointment and demoralisation (Adhikari 2013; Charsley 2008). Despite all this, they continue to hope that they will obtain better jobs in the future and improve their socio-economic status.

Many Nepali Diaspora support organisations have emerged in the UK recently; however, those Nepalis living in rural areas have not benefited greatly. Many nurses were moving around regularly in search of better social support and job opportunities. Despite facing many difficulties, they were not ready yet to return to Nepal for a number of reasons including *Beijet*, the loss of face and failed aspirations, or the overall feeling of being 'trapped' by their dreams.

Chapter 6 summarises the main findings and discusses policy issues, including nurse out-migration and its impact on professional nursing in Nepal. It focuses specifically on nurse education, the labour market, and leadership in nursing and service provision. There is a serious shortage of experienced academic faculty members as well as senior nurse managers in Nepal. International nurse migration has undermined nurse education in Nepal because the nursing curriculum has been revamped in line with the credentials demanded by western countries.

International nurse migration has had a major impact in Britain too. Ethical issues have been raised and, to deal with this, the 'Code of Practice for the International Recruitment of Healthcare Professionals' was developed by the Department of Health in England (DoH 1999; 2001; 2004). This guideline has created numerous loopholes in international nurse recruitment practice. This legislation, combined with tougher NMC registration regulation and tighter border controls regarding work permits for internationally educated health workers, has only created and fostered space for brokers to operate in a semi-legal market. As a consequence, the majority of vulnerable Nepali migrant nurses are forced into private sector nursing homes, long-term care settings, working essentially in the least desired aspect of nursing, and this has created a different professional class within the nursing profession (Smith & Mackintosh 2007).

This chapter closes with a brief examination of anxieties around the current nursing labour market in Nepal and the UK. Since the brexit referendum of 2016, there have been further complications in the UK labour market. Brexit-related debate is dominating the British political scene, and it has been an extremely unsettling time for EU migrants already in the UK. Their feelings of vulnerability have escalated, given their fears of potential job insecurities and uncertainty about their citizenship and legal rights to remain in the UK. As a result, in the past two years the UK's nursing workforce has decreased (NMC 2018). What will happen to migrant nurses working in Britain, and to the healthcare and social care systems in which they are employed, is of grave concern, not least because of all the vulnerable or sick people who will suffer if there is a lack of people to care for them.

Notes

1 The names of all individuals in this book have been changed to protect their identity, with the exception of those of some public figures.
2 Personal communication with Rita, Kathmandu, Nepal, November 2008.
3 This number is cumulative, includes all the nurses ever registered in NNC. There is no separate record for those who have retired and also those who have migrated internationally. http://nnc.org.np/#, accessed on 6/4/2019.
4 This is a short-term conversion course for overseas-educated nurses under supervision. Upon satisfactory completion of this, the supervisor will recommend full registration with the NMC, so nurses can become fully licensed practitioners in the UK.
5 The NMC is the professional regulatory body for nurses, midwives and health visitors. Registration is mandatory to work as a professional practitioner. This is further discussed in Chapter 3.
6 Except for a brief period in 1986, when 10 per cent of staff nurse training places were allocated for male students. In 1992 nursing reverted to a female-only profession.

1 Professional nursing education and the labour market situation in contemporary Nepal

This chapter provides a detailed description of professional nursing in Nepal, mainly in relation to the political economy of nursing education and the nursing labour market situation. It begins by briefly tracing the history of nurse education, charting its development up to the present day. This is discussed in three stages: first, the period of time before 1951, before the establishment of professional education; then between 1951 and 1990 as the period of establishment and professional development; and finally the period of privatisation and the rapid expansion of education capacity, which began after the *Jana Andolan* in the 1990s and continues to the present day.

There have been many changes within the profession since the 1990s. Nursing has become an increasingly attractive profession for young women and their families. For many, it has been seen as a means to accessing international jobs. With a consequent necessary expansion in education capacity, increasing numbers of new stakeholders are emerging every year. Nurse education has become a private sector business, with many seeing potentially lucrative opportunities. After an exploration of its political economy, the chapter will examine professional regulation and the current labour market situation in Nepal.

Evolution and development of the profession

Nursing in Nepal before 1951

To date, there are only a few written histories of nursing in Nepal. *Nurses Were Needed at the 'Top of the World* by Maxwell with Sinha, published in 2004, and *History of Nursing in Nepal* published by the Nursing Association of Nepal (NAN) in 2002 are the two major accounts. Some other pieces of literature mention nursing within the broader context of the introduction of western medicine in Nepal. Apart from these, there has been very little empirical study exploring the history of nursing in Nepal. This section draws heavily on these accounts, and is supplemented by interviews with some of the early nurses and other key informants who lived through those times.

The available literature, and other accounts, suggest that the history of Nepal's nursing profession is intertwined with the emergence of western allopathic medicine. The first official state-run allopathic medical services for the general public in Nepal were sited in Bir Hospital in Kathmandu, established in 1890 by the Rana prime minister, as a noble work. At that time, the royal family and a few upper-class social elites had their own health and personal care providers: personal attendants and nannies, private western-trained medical doctors and locally trained Ayurvedic practitioners (Dixit 2005; Liechty 1997).

Bir Hospital began with 15 in-patient beds for male patients and a dispensary. Some years later, though the exact date is not clear, 15 more beds were added for female patients. It was run by dressers (because they were trained to change wound dressings), and compounders (as they were trained to dispense medicine) and all of them were men. According to published works on the history of nursing and medical services in Nepal (NAN 2002; Maxwell with Sinha 2004; Dixit 2005), there were still no female staff caring for the patients there 38 years later. Whether any female patient attended the hospital for healthcare is unknown.

The first reference to nurses in Nepal was in 1928, when the Rana rulers perceived the need for female staff. Four Nepali women were sent to India for midwifery training, accompanied by their male guardians, because it was not socially acceptable for women to travel on their own (Maxwell with Sinha 2004; NAN 2002). They completed their 18-month training and, on their return to Nepal in 1930, were posted to work in Bir Hospital in the female ward – a very first ward for women in the country. Over the next few years more women travelled to India for similar training.

In 1933, the Civil Medical College was established at Bir Hospital to train dressers and compounders. Nine women were enrolled in the first cohort. The qualification or level of education required for this training is not cited in the published literature. A number of these women were also later sent to India for midwifery training and, when they returned to Kathmandu, they were posted to the Bir Hospital as the previous midwives had been. At that time the staff comprised locally trained dressers and compounders, India-trained midwives and staff from West Bengal, India (present-day Bangladesh) (Dixit 2005; Maxwell with Sinha 2004).

Period of establishment and early development: 1951–1990

Professional nursing education only began in Nepal in the mid-1950s after the major political changes of 1951. Following the end of the Rana regime and their self-imposed isolation, the new government of Nepal, led then by the late King Tribhuwan, adopted a more liberal attitude towards national development. The government opened its doors to foreign assistance. For the history of nursing, the missionary presence was particularly important. Christian missionaries, already working in neighbouring India, 'preaching, teaching and healing', were then allowed to come to Nepal to help the new government develop healthcare and other infrastructures, such as road and schools (Harper 2009; Lindell 1997). In this period, nurse education programmes were established and gradually upgraded and expanded, initially all under the auspices of the Ministry of Health and later (from 1972) under the state-run Tribhuwan University (TU), and all were heavily subsidised by the state.

A key event in 1951 was the arrival in Nepal of the US administrator, Mr Paul Rose, accompanied by his pregnant wife. Finding no qualified midwife (who would meet their expatriate standard and lifestyle) to assist his wife during birth, he requested an experienced western-trained midwife from the British High Commission in Delhi, India (Maxwell with Sinha 2004; NAN 2002). A midwife, Ms Junita Owen, was sent to Kathmandu to assist the Roses during the birth of their baby. Ms Owen felt that there was a pressing need to start training nurses and midwives in the country and made a recommendation to His Majesty's Government of Nepal and the World Health Organisation (WHO) to set up a nursing and midwifery training programme. The Government agreed to this request and, in 1954, the WHO sent two British nurses to Kathmandu to make all necessary preparations (Maxwell with Sinha 2004; NAN 2002). Training of the first cohort of nurses began in 1956. Later another nurse/midwife joined the team from Canada to teach midwifery; she was employed by the US Agency for International Development (USAID). The three foreign nurse/midwives and their three Nepali counterparts started the training in a rented house in Chhetrapati, Kathmandu.[1]

As Maxwell with Sinha (2004) states, Doctor Bethel Fleming with a team of three nurses, all Christian missionaries at the time working in India, also came to Nepal. The Government granted them permission to begin medical work in the country. The United Mission to Nepal (UMN) was established and began offering health services in 1953. In the first instance it was in the form of maternal and child health clinics in the Kathmandu valley. In 1956, UMN set up a hospital in Shanta Bhawan, an old Rana palace they had rented (Cooley 1982). They started providing health services and, in need of assistants, decided to offer on-the-job training to suitably educated local people. In 1957 two men and a woman were selected for a three-year training course, and on completion were awarded 'Hospital Certificates'.

In January 1959, Margaret Fleming, a missionary nurse who had previously worked in India, set up the Shanta Bhawan Hospital (SBH) School of Nursing, located first in Surendra Bhawan, but which later moved to Nir Bhawan, next to the Shanta Bhawan Hospital. However, initially, most students attending the SBH School of Nursing were from Darjeeling and Kalimpong in India (Maxwell with Sinha 2004).

The HMG School of Nursing and SBH School of Nursing remained the only two institutions for training nurses until the mid-1980s (Maxwell with Sinha 2004; Thakur 1999). Both programmes had a very challenging start, and for decades there were very few suitably qualified Nepali women willing to join the profession. First, there were only very small numbers of educated women in Nepal, most of whom were from the Kathmandu valley or other major urban centres. Education for women was a luxury for urban elites and affluent families at that time. There was no intention to equip women to work outside their families and become economically independent. Second, mobility was a major issue, even for educated women and their families. The vast majority of parents would not be accustomed to the idea of their daughter leaving home and moving to somewhere else for any formal education or training or to work as a nurse.[2] So, for great numbers of people, education for girls was not available and there was deemed no need to educate a daughter for a career outside of their own family affairs. Additionally, for many people, nursing and a modern western-style healthcare service was an alien concept, as they did not have any exposure and access to modern healthcare services, in rural as well as in urban areas. These simply did not exist in the most remote districts until the mid-1980s.

To make matters worse, hospital-related work, particularly assisting a woman while giving birth and helping a sick and dying person, were considered culturally polluting (*Jutho*) for high-caste Hindus (KC 2004). In many instances, some types of illness (such as tuberculosis, leprosy and cholera) were highly stigmatised. Touching sick people, particularly those from lower castes, and caring for them was not therefore considered desirable. Accepting food cooked or prepared by any outsider, and transporting cooked food around was, and still is, ritually unacceptable for many high-caste Hindus. Even just spending time in the hospital, outside of one's own home, was considered ritually unclean. After any length of hospital stay, or spending any length of time outside their community, many people would perform a ritual cleansing ceremony before re-entering their own home, and at least have *Soon-pani Chharne* (a sprinkling of gold-dipped water) to become ritually clean and socially acceptable (or *Chokho*) again (KC 2004; Liechty 1997).

Nurses from the early days further recount that nurse training in Nepal did not attract many candidates because nurses wore white uniforms, the colour worn by Hindu widows, and therefore considered inauspicious. This highlights the complex socio-cultural context that made finding candidates for nurse training a challenge for the training authority. Mrs L. Amatya, a counterpart of the very early WHO nurses, shared her experience. She said:

> I was born and brought up in Darjeeling and went to Calcutta Medical College for nursing training. I met my husband there; we got married and came to Kathmandu. My husband was then working in the Royal Palace. When there was a chance for me to work with the WHO nurses, my mother-in-law said no, I should not work as a nurse and I should not wear a white sari. White is a colour worn by Hindu widows. My husband was still alive, and so it seemed very inauspicious. My mother-in-law was very unhappy, she said, 'My son is alive and you should not wear a white Sari.'

In the HMG School of Nursing, almost all the early candidates were from the Kathmandu valley, whilst the SBH School of Nursing, as already mentioned above, received many of its candidates from Darjeeling and Kalimpong, India, as finding candidates in Nepal proved to be a major challenge. As Maxwell with Sinha (2004: 17) report, nurse trainers had to search for suitable candidates: 'UMN had issued a call for workers in their new hospital to the Christian community across their eastern border in Darjeeling and Kalimpong India.'

There were no particular selection or recruitment criteria. Any woman, with at least eight years of schooling, or who could read and write well enough and was interested in joining the training, and had her family's permission to do so, would gain a place. The nurse trainers had to negotiate with candidates' parents (or guardians), and reassure them that it would be safe for their young daughters to join the nursing programme and stay in student hostels (Maxwell with Sinha 2004). This was not easy, as the foreign nurses did not speak Nepali, and the local young women did not speak English, so Nepali counterparts (available only in the HMG School of Nursing) were required to act as translators for the whole process.[3]

When nurse training began, there were only ten to 12 students in each group in the HMG School of Nursing and six to seven in the SBH School of Nursing (NAN 2002). The intake of both schools was sporadic and opportunistic in nature. For example, three candidates who began training in the second cohort of trainees in the HMG School of Nursing were later amalgamated with the first group. In the next cohort there were ten candidates. A senior nurse from this third group in the HMG School of Nursing explained:[4]

> I was interviewed for the training, and they told me that I was successful in the interview but had to wait until there were enough candidates to make a group. I waited and waited for that. It took them a full six months to get ready and start the programme. I was so worried; I came from outside Kathmandu and was staying in our family friend's house for six months.

A senior nurse, who was in the second cohort at the SBH School of Nursing, verified this. She revealed that the nurse trainer toured districts outside the valley in a helicopter, as a part of a national campaign to attract young women to join nursing.[5]

These first groups of nurses trained in Nepal qualified in 1960. Training institutions were not only responsible for preparing nurses themselves, but also for the complete wellbeing and security of all trainees. Developing this broader security for the trainee nurses was one way that these institutions attempted to persuade families that the profession was an acceptable one into which to send their daughters. Mrs Joshi, a senior nurse, who was a student in the third group, commented:[6]

It used to be like a contract between the parents and the training authority that parents send their daughter for training, and in return, the training authority would provide them with a safe and protective environment. All student nurses had to stay in a hostel with no access for any outsiders and their letters were censored to make sure that they were not having communication with anybody [particularly men] outside their families.

In the 1960s, as part of the national development programme during the *Panchayat* era, the Government encouraged the education of all children, including girls. Gradually more girls, particularly from urban areas, but also some from district centres, started attending schools. Slowly female literacy rates began to rise. This had a major impact on nurse education. After the first few groups of qualified nurses entered general employment there were significant changes in people's perceptions. Mrs Joshi recollected her early experiences:

These early nurses were deemed *smarter* [meaning more intelligent] than ordinary women in Nepali society, and they had relatively good earnings. Even during the training period we would get some pocket money, and we started getting opportunities to go to foreign countries for further training.

Mrs Joshi qualified in 1962 and in 1963 she was given a scholarship for further Public Health training in Beirut.[7] Many of these early nurses obtained scholarships to study abroad and later received very respectable positions in the Ministry of Health.

By the 1970s, the number of young women completing School Leaving Certificate (SLC) level education increased further and more women, and their families, became interested in nursing. The few existing training programmes of the time began to receive better-educated candidates, and to have some choice for selection. Until 1972, the Ministry of Health was responsible for nurse training, at which point it was transferred to being under the umbrella of Tribhuwan University (TU), and under the direction of the Ministry of Education (Maxwell with Sinha 2004; NAN 2002). As a consequence, nursing moved from requiring vocational training to requiring university-level education, with nurses qualifying at proficiency certificate level (PCL).

Another significant event in the mid-1970s was that HRH Princess Prekchhaya enrolled as a student nurse. This further boosted many people's interest in, and respect for, the profession, given that it was now one that could be considered even by the royal family, in addition to it requiring a university degree.

By the 1980s the professional nursing service, and the modern health service in general, was becoming more socially accepted, but there were still only two Staff Nurse (SN – also known as PCL) education programmes in the country, with the capacity to educate 50 nurses a year. By this time, there were five Auxiliary Nurse Midwife (ANM) extension campuses in the districts.[8] In the late 1980s these were then upgraded to SN programmes, as part of an improvement programme to raise professional nursing standards. At the end of 1989, ANM programmes were upgraded and six SN (or PCL) programmes existed across the country: at Maharajgunj, Pokhara, Nepalgunj, Birgunj, Biratnagar and Lalitpur nursing campuses. The first college had by now become the 'mother campus', run by TU IOM, and was based in Maharajgunj, Kathmandu. The second college, which was known as the SBH School of Nursing, became Lalitpur Nursing Campus, which was independent administratively and financially supported by the UMN, but has been academically under the direction of TU since 1972.

The period of privatisation and rapid expansion of the profession: post-1990s **Jana Andolan**

Professional nursing has transformed rapidly since the 1990s. Although the idea of privatisation emerged in the late 1980s, it remained in the background until the establishment of the Council for Technical Education and Vocational Training (CTEVT) in 1989, which introduced the private sector into technical education provision. As a result of privatisation, since the 1990s there has been a rapid, and indeed a phenomenal, increase in the number of private colleges and the types of nursing programmes. Currently, in 2018–2019, six levels of nurse education are available in Nepal: from ANM training to a doctoral degree in nursing. A brief outline of each of these is provided below.

1   *The Auxiliary Nurse Midwife (ANM).* In the late 1960s, when the courses began, any young woman with a grade 8 pass from school could apply for this two-year, state-run training course. Many, without the requisite SLC pass for staff nurse training, realised that an ANM qualification conferred eligibility. Indeed many senior nurses in Nepal travelled this very route to their current positions. There were only five ANM programmes in the country in the early 1980s, all under TU. Taken over by the CTEVT in the 1990s, the number increased to 49 countrywide, and this is still the case today with over half of the institutions in Kathmandu. Employment opportunities for ANMs are available throughout the hills in rural areas, as well as in urban areas. The entry requirements for ANM training rose to an SLC pass, when responsibility for the training was transferred to the CTEVT. The SLC was renamed as Secondary Education Examination (or SEE) in 2018.

2   *The Proficiency Certificate Level in Nursing (PCL) or Staff Nurse.* Prior to the establishment of the CTEVT, there were six staff nurse campuses in Nepal, as above identified, all under the purview of TU, training a total of just over 250 nurses per year. The idea was to train enough staff nurses for the district centre hospitals, and other government hospitals,

throughout the country. This was consequent upon a review of the nursing curriculum in 1987, and the need to include primary healthcare concepts in nursing training (Thakur 1999). Currently, in 2019, an estimated 120 PCL nursing courses are available, the majority of which are run by the CTEVT.

3   *Bachelor of Science in Nursing (B.Sc. Nursing)*. A total of 50 programmes in the country have received university affiliation, currently. The first B.Sc. nursing programme was started at the BP Koirala Institute of Health Sciences (BPKIHS) in Dharan in 1993 and remained the only one for over a decade. Attached to BPKISH, the intake was only ten students a year. The training hospital employed most of the early graduates, with others employed by national nurse training institutions. In the decade following, as the private sector in Nepal started to become more involved in health workforce training, more B.Sc. nurse training programmes opened. These courses are four-year courses, and are accessible only through ten (or SEE) plus two years in science from school.[9] The rationale for these courses is to produce nurses better versed in science and, in part, to allow nursing as a profession to compete with medicine.

4   *Bachelor in Nursing (BN)*. The route to this level of training is with a year of working experience after completion of PCL training. This degree used to be run by TU IOM, having started in 1976. Currently, in 2018–2019, there are 45 programmes offering BN courses. In recent years, this course has been renamed as BNs (Bachelors in Nursing Science) and currently is in the process of being made a three-year programme.

5   *Master's in Nursing (MN)*: This is a three-year programme. By the end of 2009, there were three master's degree programmes in nursing available in Nepal: in TU, IOM Maharajgunj (programme started in 1996), in BPKIHS, Dharan (as from 2008) and finally at Lalitpur Nursing Campus (from 2009). This number has risen to ten in 2019. The course is aimed at those who want to teach, for which plenty of opportunities are emerging.

6   *Ph.D. in Nursing*: the programme began in 2012, in MNC, with an intake of two students per year.

This book focuses mainly on SN and BN courses (the latter as post-basic training) and the recently designed B.Sc. nursing programmes, and discusses these two streams of nurse education. These programmes have been designed with the purpose of equipping nurses with qualifications, not just for nursing in Nepal, but also with international job opportunities in mind. As we shall see, these have been the fastest growing programmes. Figure 1.1 shows the growing trend of nursing education programmes from 1990 onwards.

The main reason for this rapid growth in education capacity is a high demand for more nursing education places. In 2007 (at the height of this expansion) for example, BPKISH in Dharan received over 1,900 applications for 40 staff nurse education places. Similarly, Bir Hospital Nursing Campus in

Table 1.1 Overview of all nurse education programmes in the 2018–2019 academic session

Nursing degree	Number of programme	Affiliation	Training capacity/ course duration
ANMs	49	49 – all with the CTEVT	Currently an 18-month programme, with 40 students per college
PCL – Proficiency Certificate Level in Nursing or Staff Nurse (SN)	120	109 – CTEVT 7 – TUIOM 2 – NAMS 1 – BPKISH 1 – KU	Three-year programme, with on average 40 students per intake; some have only 50 per cent enrolment per year (20 students), depending on the availability of a clinical placement facility
B.Sc. Nursing	50	10 – TUIOM 1 – BPKISH 31 – PU 2 – PKHU 6 – KU	Four-year programme with 20 students per year per programme
Bachelor's in Nursing (BN)	45	1 – BPKISH 2 – NAMS 12 – TUIOM 3 – KU 27 – PU	Two- to three-year programme. Student numbers vary according to college capacity
MN	10	6 – TUIOM 1 – BPKIHS 2 – NAMS 1 – PKHU	Two-year programme, with varying student intake numbers per year, according to training capacity. MNC intake in 2018 was 21 students
Ph.D.	1	1 – TUIOM	Three-year programme, with two students per year.[10] Offered by MNC

Source: Data gathered during the research fieldwork

Notes: CTEVT = Centre for Technical Education and Vocational Training; TUIOM = Tribhuwan University, Institute of Medicine; NAMS = National Academy of Medical Sciences; PU = Purwanchal University; BPKISH = BP Koirala Memorial Institute of Science and Health; PKHU = Pokhara University; KU = Kathmandu University; MNC= Maharajgunj Nursing Campus

Table 1.2 Growth of nursing education programmes: SN, BN, and B.Sc., 1991–2019

Year	SN	BN	B.Sc
1989	5	1	0
1999	14	2	1
2009	39	14	17
2019	120	45	50

Source: Research fieldwork data

Kathmandu received over 3,000 applications for 40 places, while one of the TU-run colleges in Kathmandu received 548 applications for 45 places. Private colleges under the auspices of the CTEVT have catered for much of this demand.

As already noted, in the 1980s many young women wanting to be nurses faced opposition from parents and grandparents, but nowadays candidates are fully supported by their families. Witness the indefatigable efforts of Rita, whom we met in the introduction. The current growth in nurse education is concentrated mainly in larger urban centres. Staff Nurse curricula have been adjusted and new types of course modules have been developed and introduced purely to cater for nurses needed for the global healthcare labour market.

Adjustment of the training curriculum to meet international nursing needs

TU IOM had revised its SN curriculum in 2006–2007 and all nursing colleges in Nepal adopted a newly revised curriculum. The Care of the Elderly and Psychiatric Nursing modules were added in the revised curriculum. However, the total education period has remained the same: three years full-time. This means teaching time for other nursing modules has been reduced. A professor of nursing, involved in curriculum development, informed me that the change was to equip Nepali nurses to work in healthcare systems in the USA and the UK. The reason for this was quite clear. After Nepali nurses started migrating to the USA and to the UK (in early 2000), nursing colleges in Nepal began receiving letters from American and British nursing licensing authorities, mainly to verify nurses' theory and practical learning hours. Initially, Nepali colleges received only a few letters a month, but by 2002–2003 they were receiving dozens of letters every week, reflecting the increasing number of Nepali nurses applying for foreign nursing licences.

Another nursing college principal shed further light on the situation. Two nursing college principals in Kathmandu realised that, in many instances, the training hours in some areas of nursing were insufficient, according to the US and UK guidelines, and did not cover some important areas of nursing needed for work in these countries: namely Care of the Elderly, and Psychiatric Nursing. They also felt they had to do something about it, as many of their former graduates were already in the USA or in the UK looking for nursing posts. Without the receipt of official verification letters from their nursing colleges in Nepal, they would not be able to obtain full professional licences to practise as nurses and ultimately find nursing jobs. Principals of nursing colleges were aware of Nepali nurses' vulnerability abroad. On the one hand they wanted to support their former students, and on the other hand they were aware of the shortfall in these aspects of nursing education in Nepal. However, they continued to provide the increasing numbers of training verification letters to licensing authorities in the US and UK. Given their much-increased workload, it was felt that the curriculum required reviewing and revising.

In recent years the scope for a psychiatric branch of nursing has increased in Nepal. It has become part of the nursing curriculum, and is now also taught at postgraduate degree level. A Care of the Elderly module is currently not directly applicable in the context of Nepal, as the extended family look after elderly people, and mainly at home. It is still the case today that there is neither postgraduate training nor a Care of the Elderly department within Nepal's healthcare system.

New B.Sc. nurse training programme

Another major development in the nursing education sector has been the introduction of a completely new type of nursing degree programme: the revised B.Sc. in Nursing. Since its development in 2004–2005 as a more scientific degree it is viewed, as already noted, as the most suitable programme for the international supply of nurses. Certainly its graduates could not have been intended for domestic supply, as there has been no clear career pathway established for this cadre in Nepal's health system. In 2008, when I visited the Ministry of Health to enquire about the future jobs for these graduates, I was told that there had been no joint planning between the nurse educators and the employers: between the Ministry of Education, which is responsible for nursing education, and the Ministry of Health and Population (MoHP) and the hospitals and organisations who employ nurses, within the government system and also in the private sector.

I asked a co-ordinator for this programme in one of the TU IOM-run institutions, as to why this degree is needed in Nepal, given that not a single position is planned for its graduates in the government-run health system. Where are their jobs? The coordinator's response was that 'This is to improve the nursing standard in Nepal, bring it to international standards by teaching more science, and prepare nurses who are fit for the global market.'[11]

With this global market in mind, starting a new nursing degree is now perceived as a very profitable business venture by the increasing number of individuals and organisations investing in the proliferating private health sector. This meets the increased demand for more nurse education places, for new graduates, again those aiming for foreign jobs.

In a meeting with 20 B.Sc. nursing students, in a TU-run college in Kathmandu, I asked them why they wanted to study B.Sc. Nursing. The majority admitted that they would be looking for international opportunities.

Emerging stakeholders in nurse education: their roles and professional partnerships

The Council for Technical Education and Vocational Training (CTEVT)

Since its establishment in 1989 the CTEVT has been one of Nepal's key players in professional nursing, involved in educating ANMs and staff nurses (PCL level nursing). This is an autonomous umbrella organisation, whose main aims are to formulate policy and coordinate with all technical education and vocational training programmes in the country. In 2008, there were hundreds of courses, ranging from the short-term, Technical School Leaving Certificate (TSLC) to diploma-level training in Agriculture, Health, Engineering and Hospitality/management areas, all run by, or affiliated with, the CTEVT.[12]

The new democratic government of the 1990s encouraged the private sector to become involved in technical education and vocational training courses, in order to meet the growing need for more middle-level healthcare professionals in the country. In 1994, after a major restructuring of the health sector, the then government predicted that there was a need for 4,000 ANMs (NAN 2002). Initially the private sector was encouraged to step in to train ANMs to meet this need. Within a few years, as noted earlier, the number of ANM training programmes rose from five to 40 by the late 1990s, with a significant increase in training programmes for other categories of health workers too. However by the year 2000 there was a huge surplus of fully trained ANMs in the country. The government did not create enough positions to absorb them all and, as a result, many trained ANMs remained jobless.[13] With no further demand for this training the number of programmes levelled off at 49.

Conversely, from 2000, the number of PCL programmes started to rise: from seven colleges offering this programme in 2000 to over 36 by 2008, with all of the new programmes being under the auspices of the CTEVT, and the number has increased further, reaching 120 in 2018. Many questions are raised. How do private colleges obtain CTEVT affiliation to run a PCL programme? How also does the CTEVT manage and coordinate all these programmes, and what of the crucial issue of professional standards?

Unfortunately, no formal study has yet examined why so many emerged so quickly. However, from informal discussions with stakeholders, listening to opinions and talks and reading commentaries, it would appear that this growth was linked to the demand for more nurse training places. No national cumulative figure was available, but as the CTEVT exam section director confirmed:[14] 'The application number is increasing every year, the market is demand-driven, and there are opportunities for Nepali nurses internationally.'

In order to find out how private business investors set up these colleges, and how they relate to the CTEVT rules, regulations and policy guidelines, I interviewed the Deputy Director of Accreditation Division of the CTEVT. He explained how a nurse education institution is awarded CTEVT accreditation in practice for starting up a new programme. The steps and process are briefly outlined below:

1   An interested party submits an application with a full proposal to the Council.
2   The Council's Accreditation Division then reviews this proposal, and if it seems appropriate they write to the Nepal Nursing Council with a request for a feasibility study and their report.
3   The Council's Accreditation Division conducts a feasibility study, according to the very clear criteria of the Nursing Council and the CTEVT, as to what is required for each programme.
4   The CTEVT carries out the feasibility study and the Nursing Council has another independent study done and sends the report to the CTEVT.
5   The CTEVT Accreditation Division makes a decision, having considered the Nursing Council's report.

In theory, an institution meeting all the required criteria receives an initial five-year accreditation. If there are matters needing improvement, the proposed programme can be given a one-year accreditation, pending their raising the programme to the required standard. All applicant institutions should meet certain criteria, based on the human and physical resources available to run an ANM or a PCL nursing programme.

According to the Deputy Director of the Accreditation Division, a proposed PCL Nursing programme should have full access to a minimum of a 50-bedded general hospital, for students to learn clinical skills. If the programme does not have its own hospital, it should provide a contract letter from a hospital for the use of clinical learning facilities, and the college should build its own hospital within the next two years. In his experience, all the nursing colleges under the CTEVT meet these criteria. He stressed that the second most important issue is the teaching faculty. All programmes should have as Principal someone with at least a master's degree in Nursing, or failing that, they should employ someone with a bachelor's degree in Nursing, plus at least five years' teaching experience. The Deputy Director, however, admitted that this is a very difficult issue for many private colleges, as:[15] 'There is a shortage of M.Sc. nurses here in Nepal. So, we have many programmes run by B.Sc. or BN qualified nurses.'

The third criterion is that all training institutions should have their own buildings, with enough physical space for teaching and academic activities. If not, they should provide evidence that they have a contract to use a building for teaching and learning activities for at least three years. Within this period, applicants are expected to procure their own building. All institutions should also have enough support facilities, necessary equipment, library facilities, and hostel facilities for students. Finally, a Kathmandu-based institution should have five Ropani of land.[16] Beyond the Kathmandu Valley, ten Ropani of land is required to run an SN programme.

Management issues and difficulties

The vast majority of private colleges come under the auspices of the CTEVT, and there is a clear policy on affiliation and accreditation of a nursing programme, but the capacity to regulate and implement the regulations remains very weak. The CTEVT-prescribed criteria can be seen as fairly straightforward, but the Council has been criticised for not making nursing education institutions adhere to the minimum criteria. Since all ANM and PCL level education responsibilities were handed over to the CTEVT in 1989, no single government department is directly responsible for the quality or standard of education programmes and student numbers. TU IOM staff, MoHP staff, and many staff in senior government positions simply blamed the CTEVT, and privatisation in nurse education, for the deteriorating standards in Nepal.

Many of the colleges, under CTEVT jurisdiction, have also been criticised for not meeting the basic or minimum criteria, or for their manipulation of many of the criteria. It is common knowledge that initially all requirements are presented on paper but, once the programme receives CTEVT accreditation, there may be no full-time principal at work the next day, and providing students with clinical placement facilities has always been a major challenge. When I asked the Deputy Director of the Accreditation Division in CTEVT about this, he admitted that human resources and clinical placement facilities are usually another critical issue in private colleges.[17] CTEVT guidelines are obviously not fully adhered to in practice. Designed in 1989, when fewer colleges existed, they might have been easier to implement then. From 2006 onwards, however, the CTEVT has not had the capacity to effectively monitor the increasing number of nurse education institutions.

My ethnographic observations, in 2008, also indicated a lack of communication amongst the various divisions of the CTEVT. For example, if an application to start a new programme comes to the CTEVT Accreditation Division, presenting a full proposal on paper, the Accreditation Division completes a feasibility study and approves the accreditation needed to set up a programme. Then its job is finished. The Accreditation Division is responsible only for overseeing whether a proposed programme meets the required minimum criteria. If these are in place during the feasibility study time, then it will be approved to start. But there are nursing colleges, as noted above, where staff turnover is so rapid that it is quite possible that a full-time principal would not be in post the next day. Furthermore, a different division conducts monitoring and evaluation, and the Accreditation Division has no further role, not even one of communication and co-ordination. A Research and Information Division does exist within the CTEVT. During my visit there in October 2007, I met two staff members in the office chatting to each other. They admitted that, to that date, this division had conducted no research and evaluation since its establishment, so no research evidence existed to influence policy.

The CTEVT has been facing a number of difficulties on a regular basis and is accused of being a very corrupt institution. Its staff are alleged to accept bribes, and to abuse their power and authority. I heard many stories of CTEVT staff 'involvement' in students' exam results. There are claims that students may pass exams despite their lack of academic achievement, if they are prepared to bribe the external examiner, who is appointed by the CTEVT Examination Division (Rai 2009; Harper 2003). From the personal accounts of many students, collected during my initial research fieldwork, it would seem that the external examiners have been paid large amounts of money collectively, so that all students receive 'pass' results. Several nursing students and faculty members said that the external examiners regard the exam period as a 'harvest time'. Additionally, when CTEVT staff conduct a feasibility study to set up a new training programme, in nursing or any other technical subject, they are also regularly bribed by the applicant institution.

A private nursing college lecturer commented:[18]

A proposed nursing college should have two independent feasibility study reports, but they seldom match. Because of this, there are some colleges who have CTEVT accreditation but no approval from the Nepal Nursing Council. But these two agencies use the same set of criteria for their feasibility study, and come out with different results.

She suggested that the Nursing Council reports are more valid than those of the CTEVT, as CTEVT staff, influenced by bribes, frequently falsify their study reports.

The CTEVT also underwent a period of internal re-organisation and conflict in 2006–2007. When the initial fieldwork for this research began, there was a demonstration every day for several months, by students from colleges under the Council, demanding equal recognition for their degrees with the degrees from TU IOM-run colleges. When I spoke with a group of students demonstrating in the Maiti Ghar area of Kathmandu in August 2006, their collective comment was that, in comparison to

TU IOM graduates, they had been treated like 'second-class health workers' in Nepal. There were protests by students of Nursing and other health science subjects from most CTEVT-run private colleges. Moreover, the CTEVT staff union had padlocked the chairperson's office, as staff members were unhappy about the appointment of the new chair. At this critical stage, all CTEVT activities were suspended.[19] Despite all these issues, more colleges obtain permission for new nursing programmes every year, and this has continued up to the present day.

Private universities, colleges and teaching hospitals

The CTEVT is responsible only for middle-level technical and vocational training, such as the PCL (SN) and lower level programmes. There are private universities too. Academies of medical science emerged in the 1990s, offering university-level health professional education courses, such as B.Sc. Nursing, BN, and MN. In 2010, there were three private universities offering this range and level of nurse education in Nepal: Kathmandu University (KU), Purwanchal University (PU), and Pokhara University.

Although managed privately, all private universities come under the purview of the Ministry of Education and Sport. All run B.Sc. Nursing and BN courses, as they are considered higher, university level degrees. Three further institutions in Nepal do not yet have full 'university' status but, having achieved Academy of Medical Sciences status, they have been authorised to run health professional education programmes and to issue their certificates independently. They are BP Koirala Institute of Health Science (BPKIHS), Dharan; the National Academy of Medical Sciences (NAMS) in Bir Hospital, Kathmandu; and Patan Hospital Academy of Medical Science.

Private sector institutions, with vested interests, have been seeking opportunities to upgrade their programmes to university status. For example, Patan Hospital in the Kathmandu valley achieved Academy of Medical Science status in 2008, and the MBBS programme officially started in autumn 2009, with a view to upgrading the institution in the future to become Patan University Teaching Hospital. I visited Khowapa Bahu Polytechnic Institute in Bhaktapur in November 2008, where they were running an SN programme. The director of the nursing faculty informed me that they also planned that one day it would be known as Khowapa Bahu University.

The higher education market in nursing is expanding rapidly but with little proper preparation, regulation and control. In theory, the Nepal Nursing Council is the professional regulatory body for nursing education and practice standards. It is supposed to monitor all developments and maintain and regulate professional standards, but it has not been fully effective. The present situation in the private sector education institutions within the CTEVT and new private universities and colleges appears not properly thought-through and uncoordinated, and the MoHP has neither the responsibility nor any mechanism to deal with this chaos.

Nepal Nursing Council (NNC) and Nursing Association of Nepal (NAN) and issues of professional regulation

The Nepal Nursing Council is a government body set up to maintain and regulate professional standards. NAN is a nurses' trade union body, which has made a valuable contribution to the development of professional nursing too since its inception. The histories of these two organisations are very much interlinked.

Alongside the early establishment of nurse training, the WHO nurses, with their Nepali counterparts, worked towards the establishment of a temporary Nursing Council in Nepal, housed within the Ministry of Health. From its inception in 1958 this body became responsible for awarding nurses' training certificates and maintaining professional education and regulation standards.

Initially, the Nepal Nursing Council did not accept nurses trained in the SBH School of Nursing, as a different group had established it, and there was very little professional communication between these two groups. As a consequence, the 1962 and 1963 cohorts of SBH School of Nursing graduates were registered with the Bihar Nursing Council (in India), as the main trainer at that time had a link with the Nursing Council there (Maxwell with Sinha 2004). In 1964, however, the SBH School of Nursing programme gained full recognition from the NNC and the WHO, and the SBH School of Nursing adopted the curriculum designed for and used by the HMG School of Nursing. In 1972, when TU took responsibility for the examination of both nursing programmes, the Nursing Council was dismantled and there was no professional licensing and regulatory body until the mid-1990s (Maxwell with Sinha 2004; NAN 2002).

Available records reveal that the idea of establishing a nurses' association began at the same time as the start of the first NNC in 1958, with the help of two WHO nurses who started nurse training in Nepal. NAN (then TNAN – Trained Nurses Association of Nepal) was an autonomous body, officially registered in 1962. In 1969 it became a member of the International Council of Nurses (Maxwell with Sinha 2004). Continuously active since its establishment, it served as the Nursing Council for many years, until the NNC was reborn in 1996. NAN was involved in professional development and advocacy work, but without the authority to regulate and maintain professional standards. It has also been involved in various professional activities, such as organising nursing research conferences, workshops and political activism. There are no full-time members on the board and members work voluntarily. It remains, therefore, a professional body without any authority.

After much political activism, in 1996, the Nepal Nursing Council Act was passed by Parliament, and the NNC, a professional regulatory body, was finally re-established. It started to keep records of all professional nurses who were trained and practising in the country. Thereafter, by law, all nurses who wish to work in Nepal have had to be registered with the NNC.[20] Since then, the NNC has been closely involved in establishing professional standards and regulations. In just a few decades it has achieved a great deal, although much remains to be done in reaching internationally recognised professional standards and regulations. To date, 82,388 nurses have received licences to practise in Nepal (NNC 2019).[21]

Professional difficulties and political interference

As a government body under the MoHP, the Health Minister appoints the key positions on the NNC Board. A common knowledge is that Nepali politicians have regularly manipulated NNC regulations for political gain, ever since its re-establishment. Although its constitution declares it to be an apolitical body, many of its board members are political appointees, and are changed every time the government changes in Nepal. As previously mentioned, when I visited the NNC in summer 2006 there were no NNC board members in place. The former King Gyanendra's emergency government had just collapsed and the new government, led by the Nepali Congress Party, was yet to appoint the new NNC board. Eight administrative staff were running the everyday business, but had not received any salary for four months, and were waiting for the government to appoint the new board so that their pay cheques could be signed. In such an environment a professional organisation cannot be expected to maintain and regulate professional standards. A new board was appointed in the autumn of 2006, but there was another change of government in the summer of 2009, and the NNC board was dismantled again and a new board established. As the national political situation remained unstable until the last general election in 2017–2018, with frequent changes in the government, the NNC board too still remains unstable.

The NNC also has responsibility without authority, suggested one of the former board members. One responsibility is to regulate nursing education standards, but the NNC has no power to close institutions that fail to meet recommended standards. Additionally, the NNC has been regularly accused of being another corrupt organisation. Many private college staff regularly comment that: 'one has to have *Afno Manchhe* or the right connections to get the NNC approval to run a college'; that the NNC team doing a feasibility study take bribes, and that the NNC has been heavily politicised (Rai 2009). It has become common knowledge that the NNC receives regular phone calls from senior and powerful politicians, generally those who have shares in nurse education businesses, seeking their approval to set up new nursing colleges.

Political economy of nursing education in Nepal

In early November 2007, during my visit to a nursing college in Eastern Nepal, a nurse lecturer commented that nursing education had indeed become a *Pakka Ghata Nakhane Business* or 'a business that does not go into loss' or 'truly a profit making business'. This is evident from the rapid expansion of new nursing programmes since the start of the new millennium. The far-reaching political economy of the nurse education business locally, nationally and internationally thus merits a closer view.

The magnitude of the annual economic turnover of the nursing-education business is not known, and this present study could not make a comprehensive assessment. Nevertheless, based on the recent increases in the numbers of private institutions, private nursing colleges, teaching hospitals, nursing homes and other emerging ancillary enterprises, one can assume that it is thriving. It appears that there is money to be made at every stage of nursing education and the consequent international migration processes. To start with, as we noted, an increasing number of middle-class parents send their daughters to private schools and pay expensive tuition fees so that the young women pass their SLC exam with higher grades. After gaining their SLC, they start the application process for nursing. Today, the majority of interested potential candidates enrol for the widely available Staff Nurse entrance exam preparation (or bridging) courses, offered on the market for a fee. After successful enrolment, there are layers of other business opportunities, not just around course fees but regarding many additional extra costs and satellite businesses. After nurses graduate there are further business opportunities to be found in international nurse migration.

Staff Nurse entrance exam preparation courses

From the early 1990s, nursing colleges began to receive increasing numbers of applicants with higher grade passes in their SLC results. In the 1980s, most nursing students had second division SLC scores but by the 1990s more applicants were academically better achievers, with increasing numbers from the private school education system. In order to select the best academic students, TU introduced an entrance exam in 1993, in addition to the prerequisite second division SLC. This entrance exam is now a requirement for all nursing programmes including the SN and B.Sc. Nursing. The exam was designed to test candidates' knowledge in English, Maths and General Science subjects.

As the entry requirements became more stringent, students started to prepare more assiduously for the entrance exams. Within a few years of its introduction in 1993, dozens of institutes had sprung up, offering private entrance exam preparation courses for a fee. These preparation courses are available in Kathmandu, and in many urban centres across the country where nursing colleges are located. The exact number of these institutes is not known, but, in 2008–2009 I estimated that there were several dozen in Kathmandu Valley. I suspect this number has probably doubled by 2019.

Intel is one of the oldest and most talked-about and widely advertised institutes. I visited it in 2007, to discover more closely how it ran Staff Nurse entrance exam preparation course, as an example of such businesses. Located in Bag Bazaar in Kathmandu, it became operational in 1995. It offers tuition in a range of other subjects, in addition to its specialising in nursing entrance exam preparation.[22] It has a very impressive website, with the most comprehensive and up-to-date information on the nurse education programmes available in Nepal. It details when entrance exams are scheduled for particular nursing programmes; the total intake; the application process; the entrance exam and admission criteria; the type of nursing programme and related issues. It publishes most up-to-date brochures regarding nursing education programmes available in the country. It also publishes a glossy booklet with pictures of young, modern, successful-looking nurses on the front cover and photographs of all of their successful candidates inside. In addition, all updated posters are placed annually on electricity poles at major street corners and junctions in Kathmandu.

In the summer of 2008, its website stated:[23] 'So far, more than 1,800 students from Intel have been able to clear the entrance test conducted by well-known nursing colleges. Today many of these students are established nurses in Nepal and abroad.'

Those Intel staff I interviewed in autumn 2008 confirmed that their business was thriving and increasingly so. Intel's SN Entrance Exam preparation course lasted three months and cost 4,500 Nepali rupees (or £40) in 2008 (a cost which has doubled in ten years, to about £80 in 2018). The staff explained that their business is seasonal. Their high season starts soon after the publication of SLC (recently renamed SEE – Secondary Education Examination) results from June/July to the end of October each year and runs until the entrance examination period, and their low season runs from November to December, until all colleges have enrolled their new students. Thus, in November 2008, Intel had just two groups of students in preparation, but they would have a great many more during high season.[24] After the preparation period, prospective students also have to pay for the initial application to sit the entrance exam, which in 2006 was 400 Nepali rupees (approximately £3.75).

During training

On average in 2008–2009 the total training cost in a private college was 3–4 lakh (£2,500–3,500) and had risen by 2017–2018 to almost 9 lakh (approximately £6,500–7,000), and this figure excludes maintenance costs for the three-year training period.[25] There are additional fees for clinical placement facilities, which did not exist until the late 1990s, when private colleges started bringing nursing students into the few hospitals suitable for student placements. With the rapid expansion in private colleges, clinical placements became a scarce resource. Some hospitals then saw this as a way to generate income, and introduced fees for all students from private colleges coming to learn clinical skills. I heard many students and teachers commenting that some hospital wards have more students than available patients' beds. National media reports have also exposed the issue (Adhikari 2014; Rai 2009).

Many hospitals in the Kathmandu Valley and other urban centres have too many students coming to learn clinical skills than they have capacity. They should be able to offer them the much-required learning support but it has become an impossible situation. Thapatali Maternity Hospital is government-funded and the oldest maternity hospital in the country, and is a case in point. Until the 1990s, students attended this hospital for Midwifery, Obstetrics and Gynaecology clinical practice.[26] Students worked in a supernumerary capacity, as part of their clinical learning, and free of costs. In the 2000s, the hospital board introduced a fee for all students who came there to learn and practise clinical skills. In 2010, all categories of students in any aspect of healthcare, be it Antenatal Care, Intra-partum Care, Postnatal Care or Obstetrics and Gynaecology, had to pay 2,500 rupees (approximately £20) for four weeks' placement. With an annual intake of several hundred nursing and midwifery students, ANM students, MBBS and other types of healthcare student for clinical placements, it has been a good source of additional income. Other hospitals in the Kathmandu Valley, such as the Army Hospital, the Police Hospital, Kanti Bal Hospital, Bhaktapur District Hospital, Man Mohan Memorial Hospital and other private hospitals, also charge for student placements. This fee, too, is borne by the students and their parents.

Nursing education involves approximately 50 per cent practical learning and entails students spending many months of their training in a clinical setting. After completing their clinical placement, nurses try to gain few years of work experience in Nepal, as a part of their basic preparations for an international move.

The other opportunistic businesses in nursing education

Even after Nepali nurses reach the UK, Australia or the USA, they find that they need to provide further documents related to their initial education in Nepal, including evidence that they have had enough training/credit hours to meet professional nursing standards in their destination country. Nursing colleges have started charging a small fee for each single document and letter they issue for their graduates. Nurses have to cover all these costs personally. For example, a nurse who wants to come to the UK would begin the NMC UK registration process. In order to make her initial application, of intention to register with the NMC UK, she would require various letters from her nursing college in Nepal. She would also need a letter from the NNC, as evidence of her being a registered nurse in Nepal, and the NNC would charge her a fee for this. Further documents (relating to her financial situation, English language test, and police report) all cost money. These requirements have created opportunities for a number of new businesses in Nepal.

The fees nursing colleges charge their former students for writing a training hour verification letter merit closer scrutiny. Before 2000, nursing colleges in Nepal hardly ever received such a request. From 2000, as the number of

Nepali nurses trying to migrate to the USA and to the UK started to rise, the volume of qualification verification letter requests from foreign nursing licencing institutions rose. From 2002, Lalitpur Nursing Campus, Maharajgunj Nursing Campus and other institutes started using this opportunity as an income-generating source. Unless foreign nurse licensing authorities are satisfied with Nepali nurses' qualification verification letters, nurses cannot obtain their nursing licences, so nurses are compelled to pay this fee. These charges are relatively low and do not generate much income, but some new colleges seem to have been established as pure business ventures. The SAAN Institute of Health Science is one example. This institute was set up with an American link, not just to prepare nurses in Nepal, but also to supply partially qualified nurses to the USA, or to facilitate nurse migration.

SAAN Institute of Health Science

In 2005 SAAN grabbed headlines in the Nepali press and also became a major topic of gossip in nurses' circles there. The main criticism was that the Institute was set up as a business venture (Pariyar 2005). I visited SAAN Institute of Health Science in Baluwatar Kathmandu, in October 2006 and met with the academic staff there, spending almost two hours learning about its history and the current situation.

The SAAN Institute was established in 2002 with a view to offering young Nepali women an American nursing qualification, known as an Associate Degree in Nursing (ADN), and then helping partially trained Nepali students migrate to the USA. The proprietor had conceived the idea of training nurses in Nepal for two semesters in-country and taking students to America to complete the rest of their course, thus giving them an ADN qualification, which would then equip them to work in the USA. The training was American in style and I was informed that the programme was affiliated with Eastern Kentucky University.[27]

The proprietor, a non-resident Nepali (NRN) came to Nepal from the USA to set up this programme. Accompanied by the team leader, another NRN from the USA, they recruited a few Nepal-based teaching and management staff. Their plan was to recruit young Nepali women with at least the 10+2 Science degree, and with a record of good academic achievement.

The programme began in Kathmandu in 2004 with 18 female students. This first group of students paid tuition fees of 4 lakh Nepali rupees (approximately £3,000–3,500) a year for the Nepal-based training. After the first two semesters in Nepal, only two out of 18 students were granted US visas to continue the second half of their training . The rest were very disappointed. These ADN students and their guardians became very angry with the management. Quite understandably, students and parents started demanding their money back. This story became big news within professional nursing circles.

These students and some of their parents contacted the NNC, the professional regulatory body, only to find that there was no record of any communication with the NNC regarding this training programme. The Nursing Council could therefore do nothing to help them. The principal, who had come to Nepal to set up this programme, had a one-year contract. She completed her task and returned to the USA. By then it was late 2003 and the situation became totally chaotic. Students in Nepal had no idea what was happening with their future education. The main proprietor of the college had to find some way out: either refund the students' money or do something about it. So he approached a senior Professor of Nursing, who was just about to retire from her long-term position in TU IOM. She accepted an offer from SAAN and started work there as the Principal from 2005. She worked towards gaining affiliation with one of Nepal's private universities, and getting NNC approval. She managed to secure affiliation with Purwanchal University (PU) to run a B.Sc. nurse training course, with the aim of redesigning the whole programme to fit into Nepal's new B.Sc. Nursing programme. By then, Purwanchal University had new B.Sc. Nursing programmes in the pipeline. SAAN became just another B.Sc Nursing programme in 2005 and started teaching students in the summer of that year.

The first group of students, those previously enrolled on the American ADN course who were unable to go to America, were placed directly into their second year of the B.Sc. Nursing programme. The new principal managed to recruit more teaching staff, as prescribed by the NNC, and began negotiating with a hospital in Kathmandu for a clinical placements facility.

Initially the SAAN B.Sc. Nursing programme had a contract with a private hospital for clinical placements. But the rumour was that, in 2007, this hospital unilaterally terminated the contract to provide clinical placements for students from SAAN. I was informed that this was because the hospital had decided to start their own nurse education programme, and could no longer accommodate students from any outside institute. Given the lack of clinical training facilities, and pressure from the NNC, SAAN was compelled to stop taking new admissions in 2007. However, in 2008, SAAN managed to negotiate with another private hospital and was able to take new admissions again. Its B.Sc. Nursing programme has continued, and the 2018–2019 academic year is in progress at the time of writing.

Nobel College

The Nobel College is another college running a B.Sc. Nursing programme, alongside its many higher education courses, which include Business, Accounting, Management, Arts and Engineering. Their B.Sc. Nursing programme began in 2006. After the first group of students was enrolled for training, the NNC published a notice in one of Nepal's national daily newspapers alerting prospective parents and nursing students that the nursing programme run by Nobel had not been approved by the Council (NNC 2006). The refusal to accredit the programme was because there was no associated hospital for students to learn clinical skills. The NNC continued to put pressure on Nobel College to find a suitable hospital in order to run its programme. Several months later, due to the lack of facilities in the Kathmandu Valley, Nobel College moved to Biratnagar, in Eastern Nepal, where a hospital, named the Nobel Hospital, was under construction, established by the same company.

In 2007 Nobel College tried to present this hospital as their main facility for clinical teaching, and re-applied for NNC approval. The NNC had a second feasibility study conducted in 2008, but the hospital was still regarded as unsuitable and the application for accreditation was refused. Officially, all new admissions were again suspended in 2008; but although the college was not formally inviting applications, unofficially it was continuing to recruit new students.

In September 2008, I had a phone conversation with the college receptionist and learned that they were taking new admissions for their B.Sc. Nursing programme. The receptionist informed me that all administrative work was done in Kathmandu, but that the nursing students had to go to Biratnagar, at least for the first two years. I tried to verify this information with the NNC, but they had no record of what Nobel was doing at that time. With all these irregularities, it is not clear how Nobel College could have received its alleged affiliation with Pokhara University, another of Nepal's privately run new universities. The hospital in Biratnagar was still under construction in late 2008, but the rumour was that the first group of B.Sc. Nursing students was already in new premises there. Eventually Nobel Academy too, received affiliation with the PU and has offered B.Sc. Nursing programmes, as of the 2018–2019 academic year.

SAAN and Nobel Academy are perhaps two extreme examples, but they reveal just how unregulated the private nurse education market is in Nepal. Some other colleges have attempted to run programmes without proper facilities for clinical practice. Yeti Health Science College, for example, enrolled students in 2005–2006, but later was compelled to halt all new admissions because it had no hospital for clinical teaching. Exposed in the national media, after much pressure from the NNC, it nevertheless simply moved to a different location and reopened the next year.

Of a total of 17 institutions running B.Sc. Nursing programmes, only nine had full approval from the Nepal Nursing Council as of 13 May 2008. The remaining eight colleges did not meet even the basic minimum required standards set by the NNC. Nonetheless these unregistered programmes had been running since 2004–2005. These cases provide evidence of how commercial interests are undermining the quality and integrity of professional standards. The many satellite businesses discussed are local as well as far-reaching international ones. Some originated in Nepal and operate out of the country and others are entering Nepal from elsewhere. As will be seen in the following chapter, some international nurse recruitment agencies create links with private hospitals in Kathmandu: an indication of the impact of economic globalisation on Nepal.

Overview of the healthcare system and the nursing labour market situation in Nepal

Having discussed the professional development and political economy of nursing education and issues of professional standards and regulation, I now explore what is on offer for new graduate nurses and the work opportunities they can expect in the country, both within the MoHP and in the private sector.

As noted above, before the advent of democracy in the 1950s, the modern biomedical system had very limited capacity in Nepal. There were only a few foreign-trained private physicians for the Rana rulers and social elites. There were, and are, however, multiple types of traditional healing practices working side-by-side. The Ayurvedic medical system, based on Hindu religious practice, has existed for centuries and is also officially recognised and available within the state-run health service. Other healthcare practices such as shamanic healing, homeopathy and herbal medicine are again widely available, and also have been practised for centuries by most Nepalese (Dixit 2005; Harper 2003; Marasini 2003; Subedi 2001). It is neither possible, nor relevant, to chart all these different services and practices in this book. However, it is important to examine the modern biomedical system because professional nursing plays a central role in this.

Since the establishment of the MoHP in 1954, it has remained the main player for the planning and delivery of state-funded healthcare services to the people of Nepal. In addition to employing various categories of healthcare worker, the MoHP has been involved in training health workers since its establishment. Although, it has been heavily supported by foreign aid, until 1972 the MoHP was the sole producer of health workers in Nepal, apart from the SBH School of Nursing, which was then run by the UMN. After the establishment of the Institute of Medicine (IOM) under Tribhuwan University in 1972, all responsibility for mid-level health workers' training was transferred to the IOM. From 1972 to 1989 the MoHP was responsible mainly for the delivery of health services, for the support of health workers in providing those services, and for in-service training for employees. In 1989 the Bir Hospital Nursing Campus was established, and a few years later the National Academy of Medical Science was set up (directly under the MoHP) to train specialist medical doctors and nurses for the government health system.

The Nursing Section, within the Ministry of Health, was established in 1954 to oversee nurses' professional issues such as professional education and workforce planning, workforce development, career progression and staff deployment.[28] Currently, the MoHP also acts as a partner organisation to the Ministry of Education and Sport, and to universities and colleges for health professional education, by providing clinical placements and cooperating in planning, and policy-making.

Nepal's administration division underwent a major restructuring after the general election of 2017–2018. The current Government promised that the federal health system would be given a new structure within a few years. At present, according to the National Health Policy, there should be one district hospital in each of the existing 75 districts. However, because of geographical difficulties and poor transportation and communication networks, some districts do not have government hospitals (Marasini 2003). Some remote districts have small hospitals and health clinics that are supported and run by charities, and national/international-non-governmental organisations (NGOs/INGOs), and some remote districts have no health facility at all. District hospitals each have at least 15 inpatient beds and normally two to three staff nurses supported by two ANMs.

One step up from the district hospitals are the zonal hospitals, in most of the 14 administrative zones, with more inpatient beds and other hospital facilities, and more doctor and nurse positions. Above the zonal hospitals, are regional hospitals, one in each of the five development regions, acting as tertiary care referral centres. There are also some government-run specialist hospitals such as the Children's Hospital, the Cancer Hospital, the Heart Hospital, the Eye Hospital, the Maternity Hospital, and the Infectious Diseases Hospital, all in the Kathmandu Valley (Marasini 2003).

The concept of Public Health was introduced in the 1960s. The main public health programmes, such as immunisation, nutrition, health education, family planning, malaria eradication, water and sanitation, have been heavily supported by NGOs and INGOs. There are Public Health Nurse positions in each district and ANM positions in health centres and health posts across the country, mainly for the delivery of preventative services. Nurses play key roles in all of these services above, but I focus here on the situation of professional nurses working within Nepal's MoHP.

Nursing and the professional management issues within the MoHP

In 1993, the nursing section was dissolved, as part of government policy to decentralise healthcare service delivery. Nursing workforce management and professional development functions were relocated to regional level, with only a focal point in the MoHP. Since then, there has been no full-time and regular nurses' representation at policy level at the Ministry of Health. Nurses, working within the national government system report that they have no clear communication channels and mechanisms for contacting people to make complaints or gain support and advice, when facing professional difficulties. This seems to have created a chaotic working environment. As a result, the NAN and the NNC, with support from experienced nurses, had been campaigning for the reinstatement of the Nursing Division within the MoHP. During my initial fieldwork, I met many nurses working under the Ministry, who spoke at length of low morale and chronic dissatisfaction. They had many pressing professional issues, including the lack of professional representation at management and policy level in the Ministry. A senior nurse at the Nursing Focal Point at the MoHP told me:[29]

If you are making any policy recommendation or any suggestion [from this research] to the MoHP, please tell them that we want our Nursing Division back. Doctors have their own Medical Division, which deals with their professional issues, but there is no responsible section in the MoHP for nurses. Who is going to do anything for us nurses? We feel demoralised; there is no senior policy level position for us. There is no hope for our future and job promotion.

The reasons for this chaos were varied. One nurse blamed the previous Chief Nursing Officer (CNO) for the collapse of this senior management post, and another senior nurse said 'it is not because the position was cancelled but [because] there is no nurse in the country who meets all the required criteria to get to this position', indicating that there is no suitably educated and experienced candidate for this position.[30]

Decentralisation seemed progressive at the time, but, because of the unstable political situation in the country, this did not happen as intended, and for many years, as of autumn 2012, there was no clear line management. Nepal's health service policy has been completely centralised. Staff numbers, appointments and permanent post vacancies are decided at central level. Dr Marasini, who was the Human Resource Co-ordinator within the MoHP, in the autumn of 2008, commented:[31]

There is no clear policy on health service administration, so these are constantly manipulated/interpreted by individuals at policy level. Because of a lack of clear policy and bureaucratic incompetence, some key nursing positions have been vacant for a long time.

Whatever reasons underlie this situation, many nurses want to have the Nursing Division reinstated, for it is their professional representation at policy level. I met nurses working in the Western Regional Hospital in Pokhara, and in government hospitals in Kathmandu, who all agreed that the line of nursing management within the MoHP is not clear. Nurses expressed concerns about retirement and pension benefits, and apparent lack of professional development opportunities. Dr Marasini stated: 'There is a leadership lacking in nursing, there is no nurse qualified to take this responsibility.'

He suggested this as a systemic problem, and criticised the dual management system in public service departments in Nepal. For both the Ministry of Health and Population and the Ministry of General Administration, manage staff in the health sector. As a consequence there are numerous loopholes and weaknesses. My next question to him was about the difficulties of recruitment and retention of nurses in the government sector in rural areas. His response was:

There are numerous bureaucratic hurdles to go through here. After we cross all the bureaucratic hurdles of advertising to fill the vacant positions, we presently do not at least, have a recruitment problem. We do receive plenty of good candidates and we can recruit the number we need. But there is a problem with deployment. The majority of nurses with good academic records, who are from the better institutions like Maharajgunj and Bir Hospital Nursing Campuses, always come ahead in the selection process. But, they want to stay in the Kathmandu Valley. This way, they don't just have a secured government job in the Valley but they also have many other part-time extra work opportunities and opportunities for professional studies. They do not want to go out to the districts. After they get a government job offer, they start using their political connections and *Afno Manchhe* (one's own people) network to find them a place in Kathmandu. Many end up in the Valley; but for those without an *Afno Manchhe* connection and coming from the rural districts they don't even get any job. There is no mechanism within the government to deal with this situation. These nurses get their *Kaj* (secondment) arranged. We cannot fire them and cannot recruit somebody else. So on paper, it looks like nurse X is in the district hospital, but physically she is in the Kathmandu Valley.

Further key factors are the lamentable lack of supervision, support, work evaluation, rewards, incentives and promotion opportunities. A senior nurse in post at the Focal Point for Nurses in the MoHP said:[32]

> I act as a contact person [at the Focal Point] for all the nurses who work in the Ministry of Health in Nepal but there is nobody responsible for any performance evaluation of nurses in the country, at least within the government system. There is no mechanism to praise or incentive for good work nor any caution for poor performance. So, we nurses feel demoralised and we are here without any authority. I am here as contact person but I have no authority for anything else.

It is clear from the above that newly qualified nurses are interested in securing government positions, but prefer to live and work in the Kathmandu Valley, thereby having the option to engage in additional local lucrative opportunities. Those in the district hospitals are left without any support from the centre. Further, because of bureaucratic problems, there is no efficient and clear mechanism to recruit staff and fill vacancies. In summary, there is generally little attraction in working outside Kathmandu, due to all the factors mentioned above. Promotion possibilities are poor, especially if one does not have *Afno Manchhe* at policy level.

The shortage of staff for all categories of health workers, including nurses, in rural hospitals is a major, and a chronic, problem in Nepal. The nurse I interviewed in the MoHP in 2007, said 'our record here shows that over 90 per cent of nursing positions in the government sector are filled', but it does not mean that nurses are physically present at their designated posts.

Dr Marasini gave a more realistic view:[33] 'There are fewer than 50 per cent of staff nurses present at district level, and there is an oversupply of nurses in Kathmandu, while some district hospitals have no staff nurse in place.'

A further important factor is the structural adjustment policy (SAP) adopted in 1985, and the process of market liberalisation that began in the late 1980s (Rankin 2004). Consequent to this, the private sector has gradually become one of the main players in health service delivery. This has undermined the service delivered by the public sector. As well as various kinds of training institutions, there are now more hospitals and nursing homes run by the private sector than by the government. Most of the essential health services are provided in the private for-profit facilities. Dr Marasini suspects that: 'The private sector employs, by the late 2000s, almost 40 per cent of all health workers in the country.'

In addition, the private nursing homes and hospitals I visited in Kathmandu had very rapid staff turnovers. There is neither long term planning nor any plan to retain nurses in the private sector. It seems to be a 'patchwork' style of management, and the government has no control over this.

The overproduction and under-deployment of health workers has produced a pool of qualified healthcare professionals who are either left unemployed, under-employed, underpaid or susceptible to exploitation in the private sector labour market. In desperation many nurses, midwives and physicians have ended up working as volunteers in healthcare institutions in urban centres, without any salary or other personal/professional benefits (Adhikari 2014). In 2010, the chairperson of NNC described this situation as *Saram-Soshan* or labour exploitation. In the past decades there have been regular media reports of highly educated professionals being employed often at a very low wages and in poor working conditions, in the private sector, and initially unwaged.

There is an unemployed/under-employed workforce in Nepal's urban centres concomitant with a chronic shortage of the same workforce in rural areas. However, the health system does not have the capacity to effectively regulate and manage this paradoxical situation (Harris et al. 2013). For this, there is a need to regulate the labour market for healthcare professionals and create decent working conditions and improve retention in rural areas. There have been some initiatives by NGOs (such as the Nick Simon Institute and Possible Health) to recruit, deploy and promote the retention of healthcare professionals, including nurses in remote areas, with some positive outcomes (Zimmerman et al. 2012).

Conclusion

This chapter has traced the history of the nursing profession in Nepal. No nursing education was available in Nepal before the 1950s. When modern education programmes started in 1956, it was hard to find suitable nurse candidates. It took over 30 years to fully establish the profession. Since the 1990s it has grown rapidly, but mainly in the private sector. Many senior nurses described the rapid increase in the number of nursing colleges and training programme as 'mushrooming', which they attributed to first the growing demand for more training places, and second the privatisation in technical and professional education and the lack of government control and monitoring (Adhikari 2006), becoming a *Pakka Ghata Nakhana* business.

As of 2018, Nepal's political situation still remains unclear. All stakeholders, such as the CTEVT, TU and the MoHP face many difficulties. The MoHP has problems with staff deployment in rural areas. As has been frequently exposed in the media, private sector stakeholders are exploiting the weakening government capacity in relation to professional regulation and control (Rai 2009; Pariyar 2005). The NNC should be holding the reins to regulate and maintain professional standards, but, however hard it tries, it remains ineffective. Commercial interest has been a major force in the undermining of professional interest.

Social and professional changes have both encouraged and facilitated Nepali nurses to go abroad. The new generation of nurses seem to want to work in Nepal for only a few years after graduation, long enough only to gain the most essential clinical experience before they head abroad. How nurses prepare for their move, and what factors and forces play key roles in the nurse migration process, are explored in the next chapter.

Notes

1 Interview with Mrs Lahmoo Amatya (one of the Nepali counterparts for the WHO nurses), Kathmandu, Nepal, August 2008.
2 Justice highlighted the failure of the ANM programme to deliver maternal and child health services in rural areas in her research in the late 1970s. The main reason for this was a lack of socio-cultural acceptance of a modern healthcare system. She found that traditional healthcare systems had already been there for centuries, and people trusted local *Sudeni* (traditional birth attendants, or TBAs) as they would normally be mature and experienced local women, married with their own children. In contrast the ANMs were usually young, unmarried, without personal experience of raising families, urban-educated with very little familiarity with rural people's lives (Justice 1986). She also highlights that for ANMs and their supervisors who were district public health nurse, based in district centres, mobility was a major issue related to their jobs.
3 Interview with a third cohort nurse from the HMG School of Nursing, Kathmandu, Nepal, August 2008.
4 Interview with a third cohort nurse from the HMG School of Nursing, Kathmandu, Nepal, August 2008.
5 Conversation with a second cohort nurse, SBH School of Nursing, Palpa, Nepal, November 1998.
6 Interview with Mrs Joshi, a third cohort nurse (qualified in 1962), HMG School of Nursing, Kathmandu, Nepal, August 2008.
7 As well as Beirut, others went to India, funded by the WHO and USAID (NAN 2002).
8 This research did not explore the training details of ANM programmes.
9 School education in Nepal is ten years long (School Leaving Certificate); an additional two years with a science major is called 10+2 Science.
10 Homepage of Maharajgunj Nursing Campus, available online at: www.iom.edu. np/?page_id=157, accessed on 20/6/19.

11 Interview with a B.Sc. Nursing Programme Coordinator, Kathmandu, Nepal, August 2006.
12 All technical (as well as academic) teaching and training programmes have to be affiliated with either the CTEVT or a university in Nepal. There are institutions running more than one programme: for example the Staff Nurse and Bachelor's degree in nursing programmes. These programmes are affiliated to two different bodies: the SN programmes are with the CTEVT and the BN with a university.
13 This cadre have no international job opportunities.
14 Interview with the Deputy Director of CTEVT Accreditation Division, Kathmandu, Nepal, October 2007.
15 Interview with the Deputy Director, CTEVT Accreditation Division, Kathmandu, Nepal, October 2007.
16 A particular land measurement used in Nepal; eight ropani is almost an acre of land.
17 Interview with the Deputy Director of Accreditation Division, CTEVT, Kathmandu, Nepal, October 2007.
18 Personal communication with a private nursing college lecturer, Kathmandu, Nepal, November 2008.
19 After several months' negotiation in 2007, the situation improved. A new chief was appointed, and it was agreed by the Ministry of Education that CTEVT graduates would receive their degrees on an equal basis.
20 NNC Information booklet, 2053 (1997); NNC Act 2052 (1996).
21 This number includes all the nurses ever registered in NNC. There is no separate record for those who have retired and also those who have migrated internationally. http://nnc.org.np/#, accessed on 30/4/2019.
22 http://intelinstitute.com/ainc.html, accessed on 30/5/19. As well as addressing the nursing market, Intel offers various other services in many subjects. The most widely advertised subjects are International English Language Testing System (IELTS); Test of English as Foreign Language (TOEFL); Scholastic Aptitude Test/ Scholastic Assessment Test (SAT); Graduate Record Examination (GRE); and the Graduate Management Admission Test (GMAT). However, 'Study Abroad' is always on the top of the list in bold letters. It claims to have links with universities and colleges in many western countries.
23 Intel brochure, summer 2008; also see www.intelinstitute.com, accessed on 30/5/2019.
24 They were taught science, English and maths for four hours a day and have practice tests on Saturdays. The courses were taught by teaching staff from nursing colleges in Kathmandu. Other institutes offer the same services for potential nursing students.
25 www.studentsnepal.com/nursing-in-nepal/, accessed on 29/5/2019.
26 I undetook my midwifery, obstetrics and gynaecology clinical practice there during my staff nurse training in the mid 1980s.
27 www.eku.edu, accessed on 30/4/2019.
28 Interview with Dr Marasini, Human Resources Department of the MoHP, Kathmandu, Nepal, November 2008.
29 Interview with a senior nurse in the MoHP, in Kathmandu, Nepal, October 2007. This nurse took early retirement in the summer of 2009. When I went back to Nepal in autumn 2009, nobody was available at the Nursing Focal Point in the MoHP.
30 Interview with the retired CNO, Kathmandu, Nepal, November 2007.
31 Interview with Dr Marasini, Human Resources Department of the MoHP, Kathmandu, Nepal, November 2008.
32 Interview with Nursing Officer in MoHP, Kathmandu, Nepal, November 2007.
33 Interview at the MoHP, Kathmandu, Nepal, November 2008.

2 The international migration market economy

Decision-making, planning, and preparation

As discussion in previous chapters has revealed, in recent decades the pool of a nursing workforce surplus to requirements has been expanding annually and, as a consequence, unemployment and under-employment is rampant in Nepal. The emerging culture of international nurse migration has made the nursing workforce management situation even more challenging. For many new generation nurses and their families, an international career move has been considered to be their best option and to be the most desirable career choice for professional women.

A nurse's migration journey is, however not a simple one. It costs a great deal of money and first requires guidance about the process and practicalities of the move, and then access to information about future work possibilities. As indicated in the introduction, there are International Education Consultancies (IECs) in Kathmandu and other cities, providing nurses with this vital information. They are able to advise about potential opportunities in the global healthcare labour market, particularly in affluent western countries, such as the UK, the USA, Canada, Australia and New Zealand. This chapter explores how nurses have made migration decisions and then details their planning and preparations for the journey.

In early 2000, the UK health system experienced a severe shortage of registered nurses, and some NHS trusts resorted to international recruitment as a short-term measure. This news became global, very quickly reaching Kathmandu via Nepali diaspora networks. Word then spread of the first wave of Nepali nurses to secure posts in the UK, and those friends and colleagues left behind developed an interest in following them. Within a few years it became the most popular destination for nurses, with many looking for any possible route to come to the UK. Nurse migration-brokering agencies sprang up with the purpose of facilitating the process. Kathmandu-based IEC agents gradually began to explore new international business opportunities beyond the UK, in countries such as the USA, Canada, Australia and New Zealand.

In 2007–2008 there were over 1,000 IECs in Kathmandu (Adhikari 2010). Although the exact number of IECs directly involved in brokering nurse migration is unknown, by 2018 it had reached over 2,000.[1] Most IECs provide information on various possible destinations; country-specific immigration policies; the types of visa a qualified nurse can obtain; job possibilities for nurses once they reach their destination and the estimated overall costs of migration. This information plays a vital role in the whole planning and decision-making process. However, I will start at the beginning of the journey and unpack why the nurses who participated in this study thought migration to the UK was the most desirable move for them, and then look at how they tackled all the necessary steps and processes.

Kingma (2006) discusses the three main steps in preparing for nurse (or professional) migration, namely: obtaining qualifications (usually in the home country); obtaining a licence to practise (both nationally and internationally); and finally obtaining visas and work permits. For Nepali nurses, steps two and three are not so linear and straightforward. After completing their professional education, nurses are registered with the NNC and obtain a licence to practise in Nepal. However, an international nursing licence, particularly a British one, cannot be obtained from Nepal. This is one of the most difficult challenges for the majority of nurses educated in countries outside the European Union (EU) who try to register with the Nursing Midwifery Council (NMC) in the UK. Several key factors require consideration when making the decision to work overseas and choose a destination country. The likelihood of obtaining a nursing licence and work permit visa and then the business of finding a job are of paramount importance, before factoring in the possibility of a long-term family move, forbye coming to terms with the total migration costs. These are significant hurdles and there is much uncertainty involved.

Decision making and reasons for migration

The principal commonly cited reason for human migration is for economic gain. Thereafter other motivations include migrating for a career move or for family reunion. A graver reason for leaving one's own country is because of war and for the preservation of personal safety.

The majority of Nepali nurses seem to want to move for better professional opportunities and a better quality of life for themselves and their families in the UK. Kingma explains that 'economic migrants are attracted by a better standard of living or by the possibility that they can provide an additional income for family members' (2006: 15). This is important in the Nepali context. The migration of educated and skilled professionals to affluent countries is widely perceived as a betterment of their living standards, and that is a sign of success for the family, as well as career success for the migrants themselves. International migration of a family member, particularly to an affluent country such as the UK, is about pride, linked to the desire to be modern and successful.

Kiran came to the UK in July 2005 to work as a nurse. She is the daughter of an ex-Gurkha soldier. Brought up in Hong Kong as a child, her family took her back to Kathmandu for secondary school education. Having completed her schooling she enrolled as a student nurse in one of the TU-run programmes in Kathmandu. In interview she stated that she had wanted to be like the nurses she had met in Hong Kong, who were usually British, who worked for the Gurkhas' families, and that she was very impressed with the profession and the possibility of working in other countries outside Nepal.

After becoming qualified, Kiran worked in a charity-run hospital in the Kathmandu Valley. Three years later, she graduated with a Bachelor's Degree in Hospital Nursing (BN) from the college where she had completed her initial staff nurse education. She secured a post running a health clinic for Gurkha families in Kathmandu. When I met her in early 2007, in Southeast England, she shared her personal story with me:[2]

> I got married during the training, it was an arranged marriage. My husband also comes from a Gurkha family, so we were brought up in very similar circumstances. Our parents arranged our marriage. A few years later we had a daughter. We were all in Kathmandu, living happily. In summer 2004 we [her husband, daughter, and herself] went to Hong Kong for a short holiday. We were away for three weeks only. When I came back one of my close friends was ready to leave for the UK. It seemed all so quick. Even my close friend was so secretive, and did not want to tell me anything until she got her British visa stamp, and I was so surprised to hear this news. Later that year, many nurses I trained with started leaving their jobs and moving to the UK, some to the USA or Australia. After that I felt like finding out what was out there in those countries. So I spoke with my husband. He agreed with the idea that I should find out more about it. Then I went to see Mr Jordan, who was running the UK/US Educational Council in Naya Baneshwor, Kathmandu. He gave me some ideas and information on possible ways to come to the UK. I started the process and he helped me to get a National Vocational Qualification (NVQ) student visa. I paid 4 lakh Nepali rupees [approximately £3,500, at the time] for his services, I had my visa granted, and I came here [to East Sussex], leaving all my family behind.

She also reflected on her last job in Nepal: 'It was a fantastic job. There were over two hundred applicants for one post and I got it. I was very happy; all my family lived nearby in Kathmandu.'

Following her arrival in the UK, she enrolled in an adaptation-training programme, through which she received NMC registration and her PIN. After many job applications and disappointments, eventually she secured a permanent post in a nursing home in East Sussex, England. With the job, she received a five-year work permit. She started working and managed to save enough money. With some help from her family in Nepal, she invited her husband and eight-year-old daughter to join her as dependent family members. When I met her for a second time in summer 2007, she was working in a nursing home and living with her husband and daughter.

Nurse migration: a sign of career success and family's pride

When I asked nurses what their personal and family expectations were concerning their international moves, the reasons were different, depending on at what stage of migration the nurses were at the time of interview. Nurses in Nepal, who were still hoping and preparing to migrate, said that it was for better professional opportunities, better money, higher living standards, for their family's future and an easy life in the West. But those already in the UK who had had a taste of British living standards and working environments, as well as some degree of disappointment and frustration, expressed their feelings rather differently, some in a regretful way. One nurse, who, at the time of the interview, was living in rural Oxfordshire with her husband and two children and had a full-time job in a private nursing home, stated:[3]

> It was all that *Hawa* and *Hallai Halla* [wind and noise, or whim]. After completing my BN [Bachelor in Nursing] degree course, I was teaching in a nursing college in Kathmandu. While working there I saw so many people trying to go abroad. I was heavily influenced by my nurse colleagues and close friends, as so many of them were preparing to go abroad. I felt that I had to do something, to be successful in my professional career [she stressed].

Another nurse, Sarita, who had worked in the TUTH in Kathmandu for over 12 years, and was a BN graduate too, was working in England at the time of the interview. She described how she too was influenced by her friends:[4]

> When I completed my BN in Hospital Nursing, I went back to the TUTH. I started working in ICU, I felt that I had achieved my goal, completed my further education and it was time to settle down in a job, and relax. The culture there was so different from two years ago, when I left TUTH for further study. Now, so many [nurses] are trying to go to America or to the UK or Australia. So many nurses were leaving the teaching hospital (TUTH) every month for overseas jobs. My friends and colleagues started asking me why I was not interested in going abroad and not doing anything about it, not making any move. I tried to ignore this for a while, but the cultural pressure managed to change my *psychology*, I felt that maybe *I was not doing anything, so I am a failure* [she said this in English], as I was not taking any interest in going abroad. A few of my nurse friends were already here in the UK. Some in Kathmandu were preparing to leave. So I had to do something too. I started the process, and here I am now.

Feeling she had to 'do something', and not wanting to be judged, or to feel a failure, she joined an increasing number of nurses leaving TUTH and many other hospitals in Nepal. Another nurse blamed this 'new nurse migration culture' for encouraging people to want to go to western countries. In almost all talks, formal and informal, about the migration motivation for Nepali nurses in general, nurses talked about the *Hawa* and *Halla* in Kathmandu in young professional circles, and of the fabled possibilities for nurses to travel to this Utopia. For this as yet unseen world out there appeared better than the world they lived in. These *Hawa* and *Halla* influences inspired many to migrate, and an increasing number of nurses felt compelled to go and experience the western world, in order to be seen as successful in modern society. As Kiran stated:[5]

> We are living in a culture that now everybody wants to go abroad [raises her voice]. This desire to go to a foreign country is so strong that we selectively do not want to hear anything negative about the possible job abroad. It seems nurses are just ready to leave the country under any circumstance. Once you have a visa and have bought a ticket, it feels like this is the time and a symbol of success. I had a good job, a fantastic job, there were over 200 candidates to get one job, with a British-style management and relatively well-paid and respectable post, and it was not enough for me. When I saw some of my close friends leaving the country and coming to the UK, I felt that I had to do this too … all the family were very supportive, as they all knew that it was a sign of personal progress. Getting the visa stamped was a sign of success for me and here I am now.

Further confirmation of this trend was received in the summer of 2007, when, as previously cited, I had an opportunity to meet a group of 20 students studying for a B.Sc. in Nursing in one of the TU IOM-run colleges in Kathmandu. The majority of them stated that their reason for choosing this career path was to be able to go abroad. 'But why, and what is out there?' I asked. Common student responses were 'for further study' and 'to become a successful person'. All seemed to have high hopes that this metamorphosis would be achieved by going abroad for a better education and combining this with a job so that they could support their families.

The potential for success, as we have seen, is not just a matter of the nurse's own pride, but international migration is also something of which her family can be proud.

Family support as well as peer and social pressure to migrate

One of the main threads of this chapter is that decisions concerning migration are not those of individual nurses but in fact collective ones. Kiran's story illustrates this, and many study participants pointed out the huge amount of family support required. Thus, the making of migration decisions cannot be discussed without understanding family dynamics, and this is particularly important in the South Asian socio-cultural context (Adhikari 2011; Thapan

2005). Nurses' families are actively involved in all aspects of the process, from the choosing of nursing as a career for a young woman, to making the international move.

First and foremost, nurses need financial support all the way through: from their initial nursing education to their arrival and settling in the UK. International migrants, particularly skilled professionals, are usually not the poorest people in their society. As outlined in Chapter 1, they need a considerable amount of money for their initial education and then to make their migration journey possible. Nurse education has become expensive, and most of the migrant nurses had paid a sizeable service fee to an agent for facilitation services. Nurses with young children would need family support in Nepal to look after their young family there, at least for a couple of years until they settled in their chosen destination country and were ready to invite their family to live with them. This has also been the case for many migrant nurses from Kerala, India (Percot 2006; George 2000), Bangladesh (Rozario 2005), and is common practice amongst Filipino and Caribbean nurses (Connell 2008).

Sumi, a nurse living in a small town in Scotland, shared her experience. Her story was fairly typical amongst Nepali nurses, and illustrates how much family support they are given at every stage in their lives:[6]

> My *Daju* [elder brother] was very supportive and keen for me to go into nursing ... He did all the initial college applications [enrolment] for me while I was still in the village with my parents, and he supported me to come to Britain too. All my family are very supportive, now when I am free on my day off we come on-line together and we chat for hours. This is how I spend my time off.

The following story again illustrates how far a family can influence a young woman in making a career choice and a migration decision. Jaya, at the time of the study, was a young, recently graduated nurse, from a middle-class family, with little experience of living on her own. Both of her parents were teachers who owned and ran an English-medium private school. As there were plenty of people to do all the washing, cleaning and cooking, she had no domestic chores. Later, on becoming a student nurse, she lived in student accommodation with full facilities: food, lodging and transportation. There, too, she had no domestic chores. After she qualified, she worked in a hospital in Kathmandu and lived as a guest with family friends. She was very comfortable there, and was not sure she really wanted to move to the UK. She found it difficult to make up her mind, and was unsure about her ability to migrate abroad and manage independently without any support as regards everyday domestic work. Her family was very keen to send her abroad, almost bulldozing her into finding out about UK job opportunities. Her father went to see an agent in person, paid the facilitation fee and also initiated the visa process on her behalf. She said she had to accede to her father's wishes, as his desire to send her abroad seemed so strong. Feeling she just had to do whatever her family wanted, eventually, under their intense pressure she complied. For her, the migration decision was more about her family's desire than her own wish to travel outside of Nepal. For Jaya, migration was necessary to maintain her family's *Ijjet* (pride, honour).

Lila, a more experienced, senior nurse, then working in Scotland, had decided to migrate due to family circumstances. She explained:[7]

> I had a job and was earning quite well but my husband was not earning much. We have three children and they were all in private schools. It was getting difficult to cover all the expenses even with a bit of extra money from some short-term consultancy work. As the desire to live in modern luxury increased for everybody in the family, my husband started suggesting that I look for international jobs. This way we can afford to enjoy our rising living standard. So I felt that I was not just supported to migrate but pushed to migrate by my own husband, so he could come here too as a dependent partner.

For many families, only a nurse can open the door for migration opportunities, with the hope her immediate family will be able to join her thereafter. For nurses and their families this is one of their dreams.

Women's agency

When it came to explaining migration decisions, 'influence' was the word most frequently used by the nurses.[8] As indicated earlier, young women and men in Nepal are not used to making major life-changing decisions by themselves. It can invite social criticism of youngsters being 'strong-willed', and 'not brought-up properly'. Because of their socio-cultural background, nurses perhaps did not want to be seen as breaking cultural norms by making major decisions themselves, without full family consultation, about such issues such as international migration.

After the first few interviews, it became apparent that nurses felt it more relevant to talk about the 'influences' leading them to migrate, rather than their active 'motivations'. Nurses seemed to feel more comfortable and find more relevance in using the word 'influence', as broader social processes and relations, including everyday social and work interactions with their colleagues, friends and families, had influenced them, and supported them, to make decisions, rather than any individual's purely personal desire. The most common source of influence for nurses was stated as being their friends. Peer and social pressure featured highly: 'it is our society in Nepal; one has to migrate to be successful in one's career and as a sign of progress'. It becomes a common source of pressure: the idea that nurses have so many international opportunities, and if they do not grab them, there must be something wrong with them.

The experiences and stories of my participants have been varied. The countless conversations during any subsequent meetings and my social contacts with nurses in Nepal, and in the UK, have been similarly diverse. One element, common to most, is that migration is about fulfilling their own or their families' material desires, and about raising their living standard and social status, their family's *Ijjet*. Family, friends and even extended relatives agreed to lend them some money to cover their initial costs. It seems like a kind of collective family investment, something worth subscribing to. None of the nurses have felt any resistance to, or restriction on, their migration, in fact quite the opposite. As some of the interview extracts suggest, migration to Europe, America and Australia is seen as a mark of real progress and success in their lives, which can be shared later by family and relatives. As Liechty suggests, 'having friends or relatives living abroad provides a window into another cultural world' (Liechty 2003: 51), and looking for international opportunities is a 'must-do thing', a sign of being 'modern' and 'successful' in contemporary Nepali society. There is a new emerging economy that supports this modern aspiration.

International nurse migration market economy and the 'study abroad' business

International Educational Consultancies (IECs)

As one wanders through the centre of Kathmandu, past the Democracy Wall, towards Putalisadak, in Bag Bazaar, through the crowds and traffic, the spectacular billboards advertising 'study abroad' are indeed striking. In the summer of 2007, at the beginning of my research, just walking along this bustling, only 200-metre long, stretch of road, I counted over a hundred IEC billboards advertising education and job opportunities in a range of countries across the world. By the summer of 2018 this number had doubled (see Figure 2.1).

The vast majority of these adverts display the national flags of various countries, mostly of North America, Europe, Australia and New Zealand; and increasingly of the emerging economies in Asia: Korea, China, Thailand, the Philippines and India amongst others. As we noted, the numbers of these IECs have mushroomed in the last two decades. As their registration with any government department is not compulsory, the exact number is not known. Billboards advertising education courses and work abroad can also be seen in many other urban centres across the country, indicating the huge demand for these services.

These IECs target aspiring, educated young Nepalis, including nurses, who want to work and study abroad. Brokering international nurse migration from Nepal is one of the main businesses for some of these IECs. Nurses are thus an increasingly important client group.

As a result of the global economic crisis in 2008, and consequent changes in the education, labour market and immigration restrictions in some of the

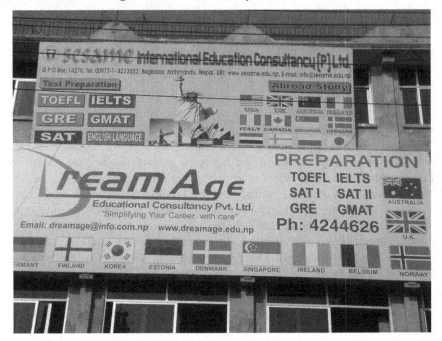

Figure 2.1 IEC billboards in Putalisadak, Kathmandu
Source: Author's own photograph

most popular destination countries, IECs have changed their business strategies in recent years, and destinations for Nepalis have diversified. However, in
terms of international migration for education and work, localities such as
Bag Bazaar, Putalisadak, and Naya Baneshwor in Kathmandu appear to be
the epicentre of the global IEC business.

There are other types of facilitation services for international nurse migration
available in Kathmandu. Some of them are truly global in nature. For example, in
July 2007, NORVIC Technologies in Kathmandu, in partnership with a UK-
based international health workers' recruitment agency called Healthcare Locum
(HCL), made an agreement to set up an American Nursing Licensing Exam
(NCLEX) centre in Kathmandu. This was reported in the Himal News Service
(2007), which read;

> During the MoU-signing ceremony, HCL managing director Mick
> Whitley said the World Health Organisation has stated that there are 4.1
> million clinical vacancies worldwide, with over 700,000 vacancies in
> North America alone. 'There is an opportunity for Nepali nurses to work
> in the US and enhance their skills on par with the nurses of America.'
>
> The initial process includes: identification of the nurses; mini-NCLEX
> examination; HCL International Clinical interview; HR interview; desire

to relocate in USA and initial immigration assessment. After the candidates pass the process, they will receive full training in the NCLEX, said Whitley. 'The nurses would receive the same salary the nurses in the US are drawing,' Whitley added.

At a time when the majority of Nepali nurses are facing problems to secure jobs in foreign countries, the agreement would make them easier to be hired in the US, Dr Mahabir Krishna Malla, director of the Norvic hospital, said.

He said the examination centre would be set up by next year. Some 25 nurses would be trained for the global recruitment this year and the number would increase yearly, he added.

Nurses hear of migration opportunities, not just from their friends or relatives, but also through reports on television and radio and social media, and indeed they can see images of nursing opportunities the west via a range of popular media channels. These advertisements are there for everybody to see, and the younger generation of aspirant Nepalis surf the Internet in search of international opportunities. Active and aggressive marketing by these IECs are further influences. Several have good international links. Some specialise in migration to the UK, some to Australia and others to the USA and Canada. The market is there to cater for modern desires and aspirations, and these brokers understand and manipulate it. Through this type of recruitment the market feeds off and furthers the migration dreams of nurses and their families.

In 2006–2007, the Kathmandu-based 'Dxx Computer Institute' offered diverse services from computer training to language training, visa interview training and other kinds of help for young Nepalis keen to migrate. The manager explained:[9]

> Nurses have very good scope abroad. They get good nursing jobs in a good working environment, good salary and prestige. But people don't respect the nursing profession in Nepal. In the UK, the average annual salary of a single Matron is up to £75,000. Until about six years ago nurses did not have to pay [a] consultancy fee to go to the UK, it all used to be free of cost. But, nowadays one Educational Consultancy named Versatile gets 6 to 8.50 lakh (approx. £5,000–7,500) as a service charge. If the visa application is rejected, they give a full refund, everything except 2,500 Nepali rupees [about £20].

In order to cater for a wider group of people, the majority of migration brokers in Kathmandu have a range of advertisements tailor-made to suit the different courses, costs and destinations.

An IEC agent told Kiran, prior to her migration to the UK: 'You go ahead, you go ahead, and there are a lot of opportunities waiting for you.'

These brokers in Kathmandu also offer 'Study Abroad' programmes and have established international links with various education institutions. Their main sales pitch is that 'Study Abroad' is a first step for Permanent Residency (PR) status in wealthy western countries.

Run for profit, and usually as business ventures, most IECs are in Kathmandu, with branch offices in bigger towns like Biratnagar, Dharan, Birjunj, Pokhara, Butwal and Chitwan. There are some small local educational consultancies, targeting nursing markets at district level, usually near to nursing colleges, offering the same tailor-made services.

Consultancies offer a variety of services in many areas and in almost any subject one wants. The most widely advertised are: IELTS (International English Language Testing System, run by the British Council); TOEFL (Test of English as a Foreign Language, required for further study in the US); SAT (Scholastic Assessment Test); GRE (Graduate Record Examination, required for a further study in the US) and GMAT (Graduate Management Admission Test). However 'Study Abroad' is always at the top of the list in bold type.

On 13 October 2008, the classified section of the *Himalayan Times* contained many advertisements for internationally available courses and how they could be sourced. That of Interface Education Centre Pvt, Ltd, read: 'Study in Australia', while M Vision Educational Consultancies countered with: 'Study in Australia, up to 40% scholarship available [a scholarship that covers 40 per cent of course fees]'. 'Study in Cyprus' was offered by GEMCP Ltd, and Friends in Collaboration Consult Ltd promoted 'Study and Work in USA, Europe, UK and Canada'; with President Educational Consultancy offering 'Study in Europe; the country and courses of your choice'. The list continued with at least ten further IECs touting very similar services.

The major national daily newspapers: *Kantipur, Kathmandu Post*, the *Himalayan Times* and the *Rising Nepal* also at the time carried large sections of study abroad advertisements almost every day. On 9 October 2008 in *Kantipur*, the Versatile Education Centre ran an advertisement offering 'Free counselling and on the spot admission', and the next day was advertising the wide range of subjects available at Thames College in London. It further read: 'Do you want to make your guardians free from the financial burden of your education? If your answer is yes, join London Thames College, we guarantee paid placement on selected courses.'

'National Vocational Qualifications' (NVQs), 'Health and Social Care' and 'Dental Nursing' headed the list of courses offered by the college. On the same page were many other similar adverts: AlfaBeta Institute Private Limited was promoting the '3rd Grand World Education Exhibition 2008', with free entry, and programmes planned in Chitwan, Butwal, Pokhara and Itahari, counselling on destinations such as the USA, Australia, the UK, Canada, Ireland, the Netherlands and Norway. The list seemed endless.

I visited a few high profile consultancies in Kathmandu: those most talked about by nurses, and those specialising in nurse migration, namely: the Versatile Education Centre, The Real Dream Educational Consultancy, and the UK/US Council.

The Versatile Education Centre, Putalisadak, Kathmandu

The Versatile Education Centre has been one of the three major IECs to have successfully brokered Nepali nurses to the UK. I visited their office in Kathmandu to follow up on their advert, and find out how they organise and manage these courses. On my arrival at the office in Putalisadak, Mr Sharma, the South Asia coordinator from the London Thames College at the time, was sitting in his consulting room. As there was nobody waiting to see him, I was able to meet him straight away. He informed me that they offer many courses in London and was happy to tell me about the Health and Social Care course, as it is close to nursing in its subject area. Mr Sharma said:

> If a Nepali nurse has at least a year's work experience in Nepal after her training [PCL or above level education], and has an IELTS score of 7, we can facilitate the process of her applying to the ONP (Overseas Nurses Programme) in the UK. This gives the nurse an opportunity to work in the clinical nursing field.

However, in his experience, nurses are finding it increasingly hard to obtain an IELTS score of 7, so they do not progress beyond this point and therefore have no chance of becoming a nurse in the UK. An alternative route is to enter the UK as an NVQ student, and this route will be discussed more fully in the next chapter. The IELTS requirement for NVQ courses is only 5.5, but 6 is better, he added. Mr Sharma suggested that he was responsible for all South Asian countries. He claimed that the Versatile Education Centre had been sending nurses to the UK since 2003. At that point they had sent about 300 Nepali nurses to the UK for the ONP and the adaptation course, and around 70–80 nurses for NVQ training. He added that they had had no visa refusals for nurses.

Mr Sharma further explained that the Health and Social Care course is about the management of healthcare, not about clinical nursing. It is better for a qualified nurse to aim for an ONP. If they cannot secure an IELTS score of 7, they can certainly enrol in NVQ training, and in this case their appropriate NVQ level would be at least three or maybe even four. London Thames College ran an ONP every three months, but the number of Nepali nurses enrolling there had decreased significantly since the NMC changed their policy on the language test. In October 2008, there were between two and three Nepali nurses enrolled in the ONP, but the college in London had at least 25–30 students in each group at that time. The majority of these nurses were from the Philippines, India and Sri Lanka, as their standard of English had been considered better than that of Nepali nurses.

A consultant from London Thames College would visit Kathmandu for an educational fair and to provide consultancy services every three to six months. All candidates' educational documents were checked and candidates could then enrol for a course on the spot.

The Real Dream Educational Consultancy

This was one of the agencies most talked about by nurses in Kathmandu and also in the UK, in relation to its brokering of nurses' journeys to Britain. For many of the nurses I met in the UK their migration was facilitated by the Real Dream. Nurses revealed that initially the Real Dream proprietor had come to London in the early 2000s as a student (his course was unspecified). His wife was a nurse and, using her networks, they started to help Nepali nurses find jobs in the UK. By 2004–2005 it had become a thriving business. Their first office was in Baluwatar in Kathmandu, and a while later they moved to Naya Baneshwor. The owner's family and friends coordinated the consultancy services from Nepal, while he was based in London, networking with healthcare agencies in the UK and arranging placements for Nepali nurses. They managed to recruit and send many nurses to the UK. While the exact number of nurses who migrated to the UK using this consultancy is unknown, nurses with whom I spoke estimated it as over 100.

The nurses I interviewed were charged large sums of money for the services provided by Real Dream: between £3,000 and £6,000, depending on the type of visa they wanted and how much they could afford to pay. A visa with a work permit for example, would cost more than a student visa. After arriving in the UK however, many nurses did not secure appropriate posts and instead were stranded with no money, no proper job, and no work permit. News of this filtered back to Nepal and was published in a Nepali national daily newspaper (Acharya 2006). The signal failure of this agency to do as it had promised caused people to lose faith and numbers began to go down. Nurses' families put pressure on those Nepal-based personnel, and around 2007, the Kathmandu office was closed. In London too, agents were pressurised and criticised by Nepali nurses. The proprietors, however, were rumoured to have made so much money that they bought a family house in west London.

Nepali nurses based in the UK also informed me that a merger was formed between the Real Dream and the Versatile Educational Centre, in London in around 2006–2007. The agencies developed a new link with the London Thames College, and with Stratford College, and were still trying to broker nurses, and students from other disciplines, to the UK for work and study.

UK/US Council, Naya Baneshwor, Kathmandu

This consultancy was mainly involved in brokering nurses for NVQ training in the UK. It was not known when this consultancy started, but it was rumoured to have closed in late 2007. In autumn 2006, I met and interviewed the Managing Director, Mr Jordan, in his office in Naya Baneshower, Kathmandu, who informed me that he had successfully helped more than 100 Nepali nurses to obtain UK visas. Indeed many of the Nepali nurses I met who were working in the UK had migrated through this consultancy, Kiran being one of them.

The UK/US Council's main link, Mr Jordan explained, was with the UK-based AIMA Services, which had networks in many places in India and the Philippines and a branch office in Kathmandu.[10] According to its website in 2006–2007, AIMA had links with six British universities: the universities of Sunderland, Glamorgan, Worcester, Ulster, Middlesex and York St John. The website provided a clear picture of how these consultancies networked globally, as well as in the UK.

In autumn 2007, I spoke with a senior nurse in Nepal who claimed that, in the spring of that year, the UK/US Council had developed some links with a nursing recruitment agency in Australia. Between them, they recruited around 30–40 Nepali nurses and sent them to Australia, alleging they would easily secure jobs as qualified nurses. On arrival in Australia, however, this was not the case and nurses had no choice but to accept low-paid or unskilled work. The story reached Kathmandu, and the nurses' families demanded their money back. Threatened with court proceedings, Mr Jordan suddenly disappeared and the office folded. This agency no longer exists in Kathmandu and nurses seeking justice have no knowledge of its whereabouts.

These three agencies by no means control the whole 'Study abroad and nurse migration' market in Kathmandu. I met a nurse, in rural Northumberland, whose migration was facilitated by the CMS (Complete Management Solutions) agency, based in Thamel, Kathmandu. She also told me that CMS has links with BSL or Blessed Service Limited UK.[11]

Clearly these IECs have formed robust, and very lucrative, links with international nurse recruitment markets. Their gains from nurse migration are considerable. This is fairly evident if one calculates the resources they are able to invest in advertising their products and services. As already detailed, these adverts appeared everywhere: on the radio and in special 'study abroad' supplements in national newspapers, and in recent years, almost daily, on national television. Via their glossy booklets and large billboards they promise they can help people to go abroad to work or study.

Migration planning and preparation: choosing destination and entry visa

Although western nursing jobs are regularly advertised in Nepal, they are not so easy to obtain in practice. There are many potential destinations, all with different options and types of entry visa, and all requiring different sets of documents and paperwork. Obtaining a British visa is one of the most difficult steps for most Nepalis. Nurses seek help from an IEC and/or help from family and friends already living in the UK, or elsewhere in the world. Nurses research and consider any entry route, be it direct or indirect, as it is necessary to enter the UK first, and then start the process of obtaining a UK NMC PIN and thereafter a nursing post. The process of visa application has become almost impossible since the new NMC registration policies for overseas nurses of 2006. The global economic crisis in 2008 then resulted in a freeze on all vacancies within its NHS. Chapter 3 will further explore NMC registration processes and work permit regulations.

Making a migration decision and choice of destination depends on the information available on a country's immigration policy and regulations. In 2002–2003, as we learned earlier, obtaining work permits or adaptation course student visas for the UK was not a problem for Nepali nurses, so the UK was then their first choice destination. After 2006 it was a different story and nurses came to the UK as higher education or National Vocational Qualification (NVQ) students. From that point, migration brokers in Kathmandu began advertising NVQ level 3 or 4 training, instead of work permits or adaptation student visas. Nurses would then apply accordingly. Others came as dependent family members, or by whatever route seemed most possible. Thereafter the flow of nurses to the UK ebbed, and Australia and New Zealand became popular destinations.

Why the UK?

Nepali nurses expressed a variety of reasons for their decision to come to the UK. Here is one such response:[12]

> I had some romantic images about the UK. I had this imagination [sic] that the UK was a *classical-place, with a preserved culture,* which I had seen in old English films. I wanted to come and see it and be in it.

For many, Britain conjured up images of pleasant countryside and gardens full of 'fair daffodils' (Philogene 2008). These images ultimately have very little practical relevance in the making of migration decisions. Obtaining a visa or work permit is more crucial. Additionally the country of choice should have vacancies for foreign nurses, easily obtainable visas and, importantly, established support networks.

Not all Nepali nurses chose the UK first. Many had tried to move to the USA and, when unsuccessful, then tried applying for the UK as the second option. Kripa, for example, applied twice for a US visa but to her dismay was rejected both times. Deciding not to reapply and having recovered from her disappointment, she went to a different IEC in Kathmandu, recommended by her friend, for advice and possible facilitation services. There, she underwent a week-long visa interview-training course, learning how to present herself in a UK visa interview situation. Eventually she obtained a UK visa and arrived here in the summer of 2005.

There are newly developed diaspora networks in the UK. These networks provide information about the application process to those who want to migrate to the UK. In summer 2007, a group of Nepali nurses from Wembley in London suggested to me that if I wanted a clear picture of Nepali nurses working and living in Britain, I should visit Plumstead in East London, and Hastings in East Sussex. They gave me their friends' contact numbers, telling me that so many Nepali nurses and their families had settled there that it felt almost like a 'mini Nepali village'. My visits to East Sussex were in spring

2007 and 2008, and will be presented later as a case study, as it shows the networks and connections behind the decision-making process and how routes and destinations are chosen.

Choosing an entry visa

The British government has various types of entry visa for foreign nationals. The choice for Nepali nurses totally depends on the type they are most likely to obtain, and on this IEC agents and other social and personal networks usually guide them. In 2007–2008, in Kathmandu, it was common knowledge that one could bribe the visa section staff in the British and US embassies to obtain a visa, and that IEC agents knew how to do it, at a price. It would cost, for example, more than 10 lakh Nepali rupees (£8,000–9,000), for a US visa and between 4 and 6 lakh (£3,000–5,000) for a UK visa. Nurses I met in the UK had obtained one of the three types of entry visa.

Entering as an adaptation student, or a work-permit holder (profession-related route)

Of the three routes most nurses choose to come to the UK, two are directly related to the nursing profession. Nurses come as adaptation students or with work permits, but either way as professional nurses. They use one of the IECs in Kathmandu or their own personal or social networks to facilitate their passage.

One nurse, living with her family in Central Scotland since 2006, informed me that she chose to apply for a visa with a work permit, although it was much more expensive than a student visa. She was not talking about the visa fee *per se*, but the agency fee for helping her with the work permit process. Many nurses prefer work permits as they give at least five years' job guarantee, and they claim that it buys them five years of mental peace and security once they arrive in the UK.

Sara applied for a different type of entry visa:[13]

RADHA: You wanted to come here to work as a nurse? Now you are doing NVQ (National Vocational Qualification), any plan for ONP (Overseas Nurses Programme)?

SARA: No, not at the moment. It is almost irrelevant now. I am hoping to complete my NVQ training first. Then I will see what happens.

Sara's main reason for choosing a nursing career was that this qualification would enable her to come to the UK. She also admitted that nursing was not her desired profession. She would have liked to be a teacher but since, as a Nepal-educated teacher, she would not be able to migrate to the UK, she became a nurse.

Sara too comes from a relatively well-off family. Her parents ran their own private English-medium boarding school in Kathmandu. She studied at this school and did well in her secondary school exam, and then studied nursing in a private college. After graduating she worked as a health educator in her parents' school for two years before coming to the UK. Her younger brother was also living in the UK. While working at her parents' school in Kathmandu, Sara found a newspaper advertisement about NVQ opportunities in the UK for Nepali nurses, and followed it up. She met with the manager of the UK/US Council, in Naya Baneshwor, paying the consultancy fee of £5,000. On obtaining a NVQ student visa she came to the UK. Her parents gave her full financial and moral support during her visa application and migration process.

Kiran chose the same entry route. She said:[14]

> I don't know what I was thinking at that time. I thought, just coming here and stepping on to British soil would be enough for me. That was my *mentality* then [her emphasis]. Jordan [the IEC agent] would say nice things, because this is his business. He would speak very well. And I did the IELTS preparation course there in his consultancy. He teaches very well too. But that was his business; he would do anything to run his business. It is our weakness too. He charged for his service, I got my visa. I as an educated person with BN, if you click onto the Internet you get so much information about NVQ, but I did not do any of that. I just trusted Jordan, that was my weakness and I realise it now. I wanted to come to the UK. There were other ways as well, but I thought this way would be the quickest and easiest one. I paid money and I got my visa within a month.

Entering as a further education student

The desire to migrate to the UK appears so strong that many Nepali nurses consider coming as students. I interviewed one nurse who came to do a master's degree in public health, not returning to Nepal on graduation. Several participants confirmed that many nurses, coming to the UK for further education, extended their visas on completion of their courses. They applied for a 'fresh talent visa' or, as it is also known, a 'post-study visa', or have extended it in some other unspecified way.

Entering as a dependent family member

Coming to the UK as a dependant, be it as a wife or family member, appeared easier, as it allowed more flexibility in getting jobs here. A new national phenomenon, this route has featured very little in nurse migration literature, but in the past two decades has been widely talked about in Nepal and highlighted by the Nepali media (Ghimire 2007). Many young non-resident Nepali men return to Nepal from the UK, the USA, Australia and New Zealand, to look for marriageable nurse brides. In the autumn of 2007, during a visit to a newly opened private nursing college in Kathmandu, we were discussing the increased demand for, and unprecedented growth of, nurse education places in Nepal. The college principal stated:[15]

> Nurses are needed everywhere, including for Nepali bachelor boys living in western countries. They write to their parents asking them to find nurse brides so they can take their wives back to the west and they [nurses] can get employment easily there.

At first I thought she was joking, but later I realised that she was quite serious and, in fact her nephew, who lived in the USA, had written to the family asking them to find a suitable nurse bride. It has become common knowledge in Nepal and it seemed that everywhere I went many confirmed it to be the latest trend. In a casual conversation with a Nepali nurse in Aberdeen in February 2008, I was told of two young men who had returned home to marry and were particularly looking for nurse brides. Two months later, I was updated on their return to Aberdeen with their wives, both of whom were nurses. Three of my interviewees came as dependent wives; one was working as an RGN and the other two as nursing assistants.

Whatever entry visa used, nurses' ultimate aim seemed to be to obtain a UK nursing licence, and eventually to work as a qualified nurse in the UK.

Preparation for visa application

Once the decision on where to go, and what type of visa to apply for, is made, IECs will take care of the visa application processes for most nurses. They will guide nurses as to which documents to prepare and how to prepare them for a particular country context. IECs will also review the documents and make suggestions accordingly and provide all the support needed during the application process, including offering nurses visa interview training.

From the records I reviewed in nursing colleges, and also at the NNC in Nepal, the most popular destinations were the USA, the UK, Australia, New Zealand and Canada, although some Nepali nurses also indicated their desire to go to the Middle East, Hong Kong, Singapore or India. However, from the shared experiences of Nepali nurses in the UK, the focus of their preparation was on obtaining a visa. This preparation period seemed to be one of the most emotionally exhausting times for them. The migration dream and its outcome would totally depend on obtaining a visa, for which a number of documents was/are required: bank statements, adaptation placements or job placements or course confirmation in the UK; *Nata Pramanit* (relationship verification letter) in Nepal; property valuation and bank details (family assets and a letter confirming family support); an education qualification verification letter from the nursing college; and finally evidence of English language ability.

Bank statements

Bank statements were regarded as the most important documents for visa application and nurses regularly talked about having a 'healthy bank statement'. It was further explained to me that a healthy bank statement required evidence of a decent amount of money coming in and going out regularly, so not just money sitting stagnant in an account, or a large amount of money coming in just once. Nurses already in the UK said they needed a healthy bank statement with at least six months' account overview, to satisfy the British visa officer that an applicant had enough money and earning capacity in Nepal, and that her family could financially support her while she was settling in the UK.

I learned that healthy bank statements were prepared in two ways. The first was to use personal or family money, borrowing from relatives or finding a financial guarantor. Any family member with relatively sound assets could act as a guarantor. All of this was done to present evidence of a nurse being in a sound financial position. The second way was to go to the bank and arrange statements with bank staff, on payment of a service fee.

In 2006–2007, in the classified section of the *Himalayan Times*, one and a half pages of adverts were related to the creation of healthy bank statements; witness this common entry: 'If anybody needs a bank statement, contact this number, quick and reliable service with good rates.'

After making enquiries in Kathmandu, I found bank staff to be involved in this complex business of falsifying bank statements to make them look healthy temporarily, and whenever needed. If a person needed a statement in order to migrate to the UK, they would contact either the number advertised in the newspaper, or an agent involved in making bank statements informally, usually through a friend or family's recommendation. The bank staff would then create an account with a large sum of money in it, as per the applicant's request, but on one condition, that such an account would be officially just for show. The person could not withdraw any money or use it at all. I was told that bank staff actually deposit their own money collectively into an applicant's account for a service fee, in the full and certain knowledge that the applicant cannot withdraw any amount. When the relevant visa office contacts the bank to check whether the statement presented with a visa application is genuine, any bank staff member could log in to this account and confirm this as a 'YES'. When the visa process is completed, all the money is returned to the real owner (s), the bank staff. The person would need to pay a certain fee for this service. It appears to be big business, with many bank staff involved in it and sharing the service fees amongst themselves. Many educational consultancies had such links with banks in Kathmandu. Those who spoke about international migration knew this process very well. As far as I knew no bank staff had been officially investigated for being involved in this type of bank statement scam around nurses' visa applications.

The majority of nurses who participated in this study were from relatively wealthy families in Nepal and, fortunately for them, did not need this service. However, some had to use this method, for which the fees were high: up to 30,000 rupees, or approximately £200–300. Others preferred to borrow money from their families and relatives or use them as guarantors.

A nurse working in a rural nursing home in Southeast England told me how proud she was of her family support. When she expressed her desire to explore international opportunities, all her family members were totally supportive. When she needed to provide a healthy bank statement for her UK visa application, even members of her husband's family came to her assistance and lent her some money. She stated:[16]

> For the first time in my life I felt that I was so important in my family, everybody, all my relatives were trying to help me in their own way. My sister-in-law lent me so much money; I felt I was special.

Because of this growing business of creating phoney bank statements, one nurse said the British Embassy's visa section was becoming suspicious about the bank statements people presented with their applications. In around 2007–2008, these documents began to be examined more strictly, and many visa applications were refused on those grounds. A nurse whose British visa application was refused, said:[17]

> The visa section staff are getting increasingly suspicious; some nurses' visa applications were rejected on this ground. My application was refused when I tried first time, they said my bank statement was false, but it was genuine. I had shown my father's money and property valuation report, but the Embassy thought that it was all false.

I met two nurses in Nepal who had applied for British visas and whose applications were refused; they believed it was because of their bank statements. Such experiences are widely discussed in Kathmandu.

An offer letter for a course or training

Nurses need a letter from an institution in the UK offering a job, a course, a training place or an adaptation placement. The majority of nurses, except those who entered as dependent wives or as further education students, have had help to obtain such a letter from IECs and some other networks in Kathmandu. As seen above, most IECs in Kathmandu are linked with private colleges in the UK such as London's Tudor College, Thames College and Greenwich College. If IEC agents were involved in obtaining these documents, they too would charge service fees.

Nurses admitted that those documents, relating to training or courses, as supplied by the agents, were often forged, and that the agents asked for the documents back when nurses arrived in the UK. Nurses who had obtained such documents from agents said they did not know whether the documents were genuine or not, until they arrived in the UK. Later, they learned that some of the colleges used to create these documents did not even run the preadaptation and adaptation training programmes, as stated in their offer letter. One nurse who entered the UK as an adaptation student through the help of one of the IECs said:[18]

> I was very nervous when I learnt that I was travelling all the way to Britain and holding false documents. When the agents asked for all of them back after I arrived here, I said these were official, so legal, documents and I wanted to keep them with me. When I realised that they were all false, I destroyed and disposed of them. I was very nervous.

Many nurses had such faked letters declaring that they were enrolled for adaptation or pre-adaptation nurse training in a college. Those who had used their own personal and professional links, however, felt that their letters were genuine. Those who had relations and family in the UK had a different set of documents.

Proof of family relations and property valuation letter

These letters were supplied in Nepal, usually by the local authority. Their purpose is to show the Visa Officer that the nurse has had family support and that her family are financially sound. This provided additional support for their bank statements.

Evidence of professional qualifications and qualifications verification letters

All nurses submitted these documents with their visa application. One is required from the Nepal Nursing Council, as proof of their professional licence in Nepal, and another from their initial training institution, as proof of their professional qualification. According to the nurses with whom I spoke, all of these documents so far have been genuine.

Finally, some nurses had received visa interview preparation training. Many had undertaken an English Language course, and IELTS preparation. Evidence of English language proficiency had been optional for many in the early days of migration, and was not needed for those who come to the UK as dependent wives until July 2010.

Conclusion

Recent social changes in Nepal, and changes in media and Internet technology globally, have created and fuelled the desire for educated and skilled

Nepali professionals to go abroad. International migration as a professional nurse is perceived as the most desirable career option for women.

Globally nurses seem to be in a good position to make international moves (Percot 2006; Kingma 2006; George 2000) and this applies to Nepali nurses too. Nepali nurses use various IECs and other professional and social networks. Family connections and the full family support they receive also play their part in the fulfilment of their dreams. Nurses tried to obtain whichever entry visa seemed the most likely, but not all were fortunate enough to obtain one for their desired destination country. Those without strong family and professional support and connections internationally, have had little choice but to rely on the information given to them by the IECs' agents, and the process became very costly and risky.

The media has frequently exposed IECs for providing false information to Nepali students and potential migrants. Stories of nurses being cheated by IEC agents have been frequently heard (Acharya 2006). The *Himalayan Times* of 12 November 2008 published an article by Subba, entitled 'Power of correct info', in which the Australian Ambassador, Mr Lade, advised Nepali students to learn first about the visa regulations and courses and universities in Australia, not just to trust the brokers, because some of the claims the agents advertise turn out to be too good to be true (Subba 2008).[19] Similarly, the US embassy in Nepal issued the following notice in January 2009 (*Nepalnews.com* 2009): 'We hear stories of unscrupulous consultancies offering packets of fake financial documents for sale or schemes involving a supposed "job" in the US for hefty amounts', the US Embassy's Consul, Mea Arnold, declared at a press conference.

When the British visa office rejected Nepali nurses' visa applications on financial grounds, on suspicion of fake bank statements, nurses were very angry and frustrated, as they had already paid the fees for arranging future jobs or courses, but the agents had not refunded them. Unfortunately, the information supplied by IECs quite often turned out to be false. However, these agents are incredibly cunning, altering their strategies and quickly adapting to changing visa policies and regulations. Accordingly, some nurses had made visa applications several times and to multiple destination countries. Eventually some obtained UK visas and travelled to the UK. What happened to them when they arrived there is explored in the following chapter.

Notes

1 Interview with the director of an IEC, Kathmandu, Nepal, January 2019.
2 Interviewed in East Sussex, England, February 2007.
3 Interviewed in rural Oxfordshire, England, February 2007.
4 Interviewed in rural Buckinghamshire, England, February 2007.
5 Interviewed in East Sussex, England, February 2008.
6 Interviewed in Dundee, Scotland, June 2007.
7 Interviewed in Aberdeen, Scotland, January 2008.

8 Nurses used the English word 'influence'.
9 Interviewed in Kathmandu, Nepal, July 2007.
10 See www.aimagroup.co.uk/ accessed on 27/6/2010. Although the UK/US Council was closed in 2007, AIMA still has a branch office in Kathmandu.
11 Detailed information about BLS was available in their website. www.blessedservices. co.uk/, accessed on 12/2/2009.
12 Interviewed in rural Oxfordshire, England, March 2007.
13 Interviewed in rural Oxfordshire, England, March 2007.
14 Interviewed in East Sussex, England, February 2008.
15 Interview with a private nursing college principal, Kathmandu, Nepal, October 2007.
16 Interviewed in East Sussex, England, April 2008.
17 Interviewed in rural Oxfordshire, England, February 2007.
18 Interviewed in rural Oxfordshire, England, February 2007.
19 www.thehimalayantimes.com, accessed on 12/11/2008. The same article states that nursing is the fifth-most desired course for Nepalis to study in Australia and that student numbers had grown by 110 per cent in 2008.

3 Arriving and surviving in the UK

Navigating a new set of professional challenges

As indicated earlier, since tougher nurse licensing, and corresponding changes in immigration policy, were introduced in the UK in 2006, the flow of nurses migrating from Nepal to the UK ebbed, with Australia becoming the most popular and convenient migration destination. This is still very much the case today, but this chapter returns to the period prior to the global economic crisis of 2008, to focus specifically on Nepali nurses' arrival in the UK.

After obtaining a British visa, nurses wasted no time in Nepal and would board the earliest suitable flight to London. They had the many adjustments all migrants need to make on arrival in a new environment, but first and foremost, they needed to find accommodation, before securing a job and starting their lives in this new society. To work as qualified nurses they would need to obtain the all-important the UK Nursing licence: the NMC-UK PIN, a process made very difficult for overseas nurses by those 2006 changes. Thereafter, to be able to live and work legally in the UK, a valid visa or work permit has been required, involving a negotiation of ever-changing UK immigration regulations. As can be imagined, these major challenges ultimately affect nurses' professional and social assimilation. Their next hurdle had been to secure a full-time, and preferably a permanent job. As this chapter will further demonstrate, no step of this journey was in any way easy. Any available support from social and professional networks and IECs became vital in those early days. I begin by looking at the trend of Nepali nurse migration to the UK and then at their further steps as they prepared to set up a new life.

Nepali Nurses in Britain: migration trend, available data and entry visa

Available records, and information on 'out of country' movements of nurses from Nepal suggest that, in the main, Nepali nurses started coming to the UK from 2000. Before this, only a few nurses came to the UK, and then returned home after a period of further education or training. Some nurses travelled as dependent family members, but the wider, and organised, nurse migration market that we see today did not exist.

Nursing shortages in the UK in the early 2000s were a trigger factor for Nepali nurses' migration. With many nursing vacancies in the National Health System (NHS) as well as in the private nursing home sector, the UK Home Office had made special provision for foreign nurses by streamlining the work permit process. Organising and obtaining a job and work permit was straightforward at that time.

In the early 2000s Nepali nurses' migration evolved through Nepali Diaspora networks and other personal connections. Just a few nurses came at first, after which many others began to make enquiries about job possibilities, and the numbers started to rise: a pattern commonly described as 'chain migration' (Ahmed 2005; Castle 2000). Gradually a thriving migration business developed in Nepal, involving Nepali, British and other international recruitment agencies.

Finding exact data on migration has been a challenge for migration researchers globally (Castle 2000; Saravia & Miranda 2004; Diallo 2004), and finding any data on nurse migration from Nepal has been extremely challenging. International nurse migration being a new phenomenon, there was no recording system on nurses' out-migration at all until 2003–2004, and there is no systematic and proper recording system as yet in Nepal. Accordingly I have used any available records, usually *ad hoc* in nature, to gather information on nurse migration: the Nepal Nursing Council register; records kept by a few nursing colleges on qualification verification issued for their graduates; the British Embassy visa section records (relevant up to 2008 as thereafter contracted out to a private agency); as well as information from IECs in Nepal.

The NMC UK is an independent professional regulatory body for all qualified nurses, midwives and health visitors in the UK. To practise nursing in the UK nurses must register with the NMC by law. It sets all standards and practice regulations, which all nurses, midwives and health visitors must follow. Registration criteria for internationally qualified nurses are also determined and set by the NMC. At the UK end, NMC keeps records of all suitably qualified and eligible nurses and midwives registered to practise in the UK, as are the countries of origin of all internationally qualified nurses. Registration records run from 1 April–31 March each year. Figure 3.1 illustrates the rising trend of Nepali nurses and midwives obtaining the NMC UK registration to practice.

NMC records would suggest that between the beginning of April 2002 and the end of March 2008, 527 Nepal trained nurses were entered in the NMC register as initial registrants; most of them then obtained a full licence to practise as nurses (NMC 2009). However, drawing on available data sources, it is estimated that by the end of 2008 as many as 1,000 Nepal-educated nurses had migrated to the UK. The number continued to increase for a few years, even after the global economic crisis of 2008. NNA UK[1] speculates that around 2,000 Nepal-educated nurses have migrated to the UK. In the past decade, however, the number of Nepali nurses in the UK is likely to have remained the same, given their preference for Australia.

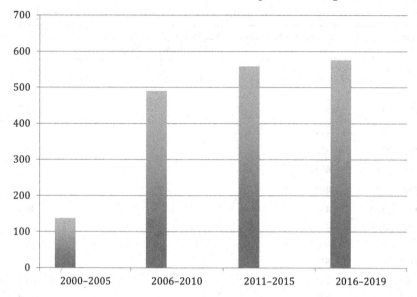

Figure 3.1 Total number of Nepali (Nepal-educated) nurses registered by the NMC (UK)
Source: statistical analysis of the NMC UK register, June 2019

A nurse's initial registration application with the NMC, however, does not mean that s/he actually has moved to the UK to work. It was assumed that this source offered a reliable and trustworthy indicator of the number of Nepali nurses obtaining nursing licences in the UK and entering the healthcare system here. However, in addition to official NMC records, many Nepali nurses I met in the UK before 2009, had entered as dependent family members or as students, and were planning thereafter to apply for NMC registration.

According to the NMC register, prior to 2002, Nepal was subsumed under the category of 'other', as the number of its nurses entering in the NMC UK had been insignificant.[2] A total of 162 Nepali nurse applications had been processed by the NMC UK, but it is not clear how many were actually fully registered and had obtained their PIN. When the NMC started its new recording system in 2002–2003, Nepal was then listed as a new source country. In that year, there were 71 Nepali nurses registered, and Nepal ranked 24th in a list of countries sending nurses to the UK. However, in 2007–2008 this figure rose to 475, and Nepal became 5th in the hierarchy of source countries for internationally educated nurses. Further examination of the NMC data in June 2019 suggests that the number peaked in 2015–2016 to 584 and since then has declined slowly. In 2018–2019 the number has fallen to 576. A possible reason for this decline could be that some of the nurses have taken retirement in this period. Table 3.1 provides a cumulative number in the NMC UK register, from early 2000 until the end of March 2019.

Table 3.1 Nepal-educated nurses on the NMC UK register, up until 31 March 2019

Years	Number of nurses	Number of duel-registered (nurse and midwife) individuals	Total
2002–2003	21		21
2003–2004	64		64
2004–2005	137		137
2005–2006	212		212
2006–2007	359		359
2007–2008	475		475
2008–2009	485		485
2009–2010	489	1	490
2010–2011	491	2	493
2011–2012	506	2	508
2012–2013	519	2	521
2013–2014	545	2	547
2014–2015	557	2	559
2015–2016	582	2	584
2016–2017	578	2	580
2017–2018	576	2	578
2018–2019	574	2	576

Source: NMC UK register 2019

Further, the number of nurses obtaining their NMC PIN in a particular year does not always mean these nurses had newly arrived in the UK. Some nurses could have been living in the UK for several years before obtaining an NMC PIN. Apart from those fully registered with the NMC, many Nepali nurses without an NMC PIN work as care workers and nursing assistants here. During the initial research fieldwork period (2006–2009), some Nepali nurses were preparing for the English language test required for NMC-UK registration, whilst others were already disheartened by the whole registration process and were looking for opportunities elsewhere.

Information obtained from IECs in Kathmandu, the British Embassy visa section in Kathmandu (before it was privatised and moved to New Delhi, India), and interviews with Nepali nurses in the UK, revealed that Nepali nurses obtained three types of entry visa to come to the UK. These were described in Chapter 2 and the most common choice of entry visa is directly related to their professional work, the remaining two being for dependent family members visa or postgraduate students. Nursing or healthcare-related visas are subdivided into the following three categories.

National Vocational Qualification (NVQ) level 3 or 4 student visas

Nurses with NVQ visas are expected to undertake Health and Social Care level 3 or 4 courses, as provided by UK colleges and higher education institutions. Unfortunately, it does not lead directly to NMC UK registration and a full nursing licence, but it was perceived as an easy route into the UK. Informed by IECs in Nepal that these courses were usually 12–18 months in length, nurses applying for this type of visa initially had 18-month student visas.[3]

Overseas Nurses Programme (ONP)

Until July 2006 this was known as an 'Adaptation Course' or 'Supervised Practice Placement', thereafter reconfigured as the 'Overseas Nursing Programme (ONP)'. The Adaptation Course was available for internationally educated nurses, within the NHS or in private-sector healthcare institutions, where there was an NMC-recognised and qualified mentor for their supervision, support and assessment. When a mentor judged a trainee nurse to be ready to practise safely, he/she would be recommended for full NMC registration. After the changes of 2006, the ONP became the course offered by Higher Education Institutions in the UK. However, entry into this course was very difficult, given the introduction of very strict entry criteria (NMC 2010).[4]

Work permit visa

Between 2000 and 2004, there was an active recruitment of nurses from international sources, the UK Home Office having listed nursing as a 'shortage profession'. Healthcare institutions recruiting internationally at that time could fast-track work permits, granting nurses work permit visas to work full-time in the NHS and in private nursing homes (Buchan 2002). Then, those Nepali nurses who had a four-year work permit visa obtained them from the British Embassy in Kathmandu. This visa allowed initial pre-registration training and led to work as fully registered nurses afterwards.[5]

Arriving and professional assimilation in the UK

Leaving Nepal and arriving in the UK

After all the hard and stressful work involved in obtaining their visas, prospective migrants, be they either skilled professionals or students, have parties and celebrations before leaving home. This is a common social practice in Nepal, and for those nurses, delighted at having obtained their visas, this last week is usually a very happy, exciting and busy time. When recounting their long journeys, nurses expressed their sense of relief on clearing emigration in Kathmandu and on gaining their eventual entry into the UK. Clearing emigration at Kathmandu airport can be a nightmare for any traveller, but particularly difficult for women travelling on their own. Regarding nurses' early arrival experiences, these seem to have been mixed. It had been a dream come true, but also evoked a tremendous amount of anxiety and feelings of insecurity. The challenges of NMC registration and professional assimilation still lay ahead.

Eligibility to practise nursing in the UK, as we learned, depends on obtaining an NMC PIN before a post can be secured. Nepali nurses must undergo the appropriate training. How smoothly and swiftly this could be achieved depended on two main factors: the timing of their arrival, and how well nurses were connected and supported by existing social and professional networks once in the UK. Most Nepali nurses who participated in this study had obtained their NMC PIN before 2006, with only a few obtaining them thereafter. As such, it is important to examine both registration processes to understand fully the changes in the NMC registration system.

NMC UK registration regulation — before July 2006

Until July 2006, the decision on eligibility for NMC registration for any internationally educated nurse would be made on an individual basis. The NMC would issue a decision letter to an internationally educated applicant, after careful examination of the applicant's initial nursing education and subsequent work experience in her own country. The most common decision given to Nepal educated nurses used to be that applicants were to complete a period of supervised placement, in a UK healthcare facility. This could take from three months to a year, depending on when the nurse's clinical supervisor/mentor felt that the applicant was ready to practise independently and safely in the UK. The placement would be anywhere deemed suitable for the UK pre-registration nurses to learn and practise clinical skills; for example in an independently run nursing home or in an NHS hospital ward. The NMC UK, however, had recognised the fact that there were only limited numbers of training places available, so nurses were advised not to travel to the UK until they had found suitable placements.

Many internationally educated nurses found it impossible to secure a training placement in the UK, whilst living in their home country. Despite the NMC's advice, many nurses, including Nepali nurses, decided to come to the UK first, then search for a placement afterwards (Smith et al. 2006). Their explanation for this was that the NMC decision letter remained valid for only two years, and so they would try and find a placement within this period. Many felt that if they were to follow the NMC's advice they would never make it to the UK.

Some nurses I met and interviewed said their NMC decision letter expired while they were waiting for suitable placements in the UK, so they had to start the whole application process all over again. This meant further payment, and it became very costly for them. Some arrived just a few months before their NMC decision was due to expire. Yet, even though nurses faced all these practical hurdles and difficulties in finding an adaptation course placement, the NMC continued to receive increasing numbers of applications from international candidates.

Crucially there were few suitable places for international nurses' adaptation training, and the capacity of those facilities remained small. A large number of internationally educated nurses were already in the UK. Findings of a joint research by the Open University, the University of Surrey and the RCN on 'overseas nurses and their career progression' suggested that, in 2006, there were over 37,000 nurses waiting in limbo for suitable placements for adaptation training and supervised practice placements (Smith et al. 2006; Parish 2006). At a time when so many internationally qualified nurses were desperate to undergo the training process, the NHS stopped employing international nurses when the UK Home Office changed work-permit regulations. Parish described this as: 'the tap has now been turned off mid-flow' (2006: 7).

Kingma (2006: 101) points out that some private agents saw this gap as a business opportunity. They began to charge exorbitant fees for adaptation training placements but without providing the much-required supervision and guidance. She further reports that a private nursing home mentor allegedly provided mentorship to 113 foreign nurses over a period of three months, which, as the author points out, 'is a physically impossible task'. This trend was associated with sub-standard monitoring and regulation of private-sector training placements.

Additionally, reports began to emerge in the British media of many home-trained nurses remaining unemployed (Hancock 2008). Simultaneously in 2005–2006, because of economic constraints, NHS employment capacity was reduced, thus yet again worsening opportunities for internationally educated nurses. In order to combat the situation in the UK, it was thought that stricter regulation was needed, hence the changes the NMC UK made to their international nurse registration regulations, from August 2006.

NMC UK's new registration criteria after July 2006: the Overseas Nurses Programme (ONP)

To this day, for registration purposes, all internationally educated nurses are placed in two categories: nurses educated in the European Union (EU) and nurses educated outwith EU countries (NMC 2018).[6] Nurses from countries outside the EU have to obtain an International English Language Testing System (IELTS) score of 7 in all areas including skills of listening, reading, writing and speaking. This test score has proved a tough challenge for many. An NHS nurse manager, involved in running training for foreign nurses, observed that[7] 'This was deliberately introduced to control the number of overseas applications.'

With the advent of these further stipulations, the number of applications from internationally educated nurses fell significantly. According to the NMC, in May 2008, this figure came down to 193.[8] During the initial fieldwork (2006–2009), I encountered many Nepali nurses in the UK still awaiting registration but who had been held back because they were unable to obtain the required IELTS score.[9]

Once internationally educated nurses obtained that requisite score, they would be eligible to enrol for the ONP. Designed to offer nurses better training, supervision and support, it comprises 20 days of protected and structured learning and a three-month period of clinical placements. All ONP courses are standardised and the clinical placements, where nurses go for supervised practice, are properly monitored as to their suitability by a local higher education institution approved by NMC UK.

When nurses complete this training they receive recommendations from their clinical supervisors for full registration as qualified nurses. Then they pay a further registration fee and obtain their PIN. From 2013, this registration has had to be renewed annually.

Nepali nurses' experience of adaptation training placement

Fifteen out of the 22 Nepali nurses I interviewed in the UK had received their NMC PIN. Fourteen of them had completed their adaptation training in private nursing homes; one had completed theirs in an NHS hospital, after having worked in a nursing home.[10] Five of them had had no luck with finding adaptation placements or ONP courses, and two nurses were under ONP training at the time of my initial research interviews (2006–2009). The majority of nurses who completed their training in nursing homes felt that the adaptation training was very useful, but only to work in a nursing home situation, and in long-term care settings. Most nurses found it inadequate for learning and practising any advanced clinical nursing skills, required for work in an acute clinical setting in the UK.

Most nurses felt that, during their adaptation period, they were not fully supported by experienced mentors, but rather policed by staff less qualified and less experienced than they were. Lila, for example, was assigned to a carer during her adaptation in a nursing home (in early 2000). She said:[11] 'How can a carer help me to learn about nursing in Britain? What could she teach me – she could not even read patients' notes herself.'

Lila already held a master's degree from Nepal, and felt humiliated and undervalued being supervised by healthcare assistants in a nursing home. She stressed there were insufficient properly qualified and experienced mentors in the nursing home where she was undertaking her training, to provide that much-needed support for her. Staffed mostly by care assistants, this nursing home had only one or two NMC registered nurses on each shift. They would have been more appropriate mentors, but she was given no other options.

Those who obtained registration through the old system (pre-ONP) revealed that policy and regulations were unclear and inconsistent. Nursing homes had no standard training criteria and guidelines. Kingma (2006) and the RCN (2003) have also highlighted this issue: some privately run nursing homes were not monitored and audited rigorously at all. Trainee nurses' named mentors existed only on paper, and many felt that the whole training programme was left up to their mentor alone. Even if not working closely together, maintaining a good personal relationship with one's mentor was vital, and the better that relationship the easier and smoother the training became. Although the quality of training they received was not of a high standard, many felt it was very important for them to complete it as quickly as possible. I also heard a great many rumours of trainee nurses bribing their mentors, with gold jewellery and other expensive gifts, so they might obtain their NMC PIN smoothly. Most nurses were just desperate to be able to apply for proper nursing posts.

Job market and work permit situation, and nurses' experience

A work permit visa is also required in order to work in the UK. It is granted when there is a direct agreement between two governments or, in the case of nurses recruited directly from outside the EU, to fill any vacancies not filled by local, regional and national recruitment efforts. There has been no direct agreement yet between the Nepali and British governments as regards recruitment and work permit provision for Nepali nurses.

Once an employer obtains a work permit from the Home Office to employ a particular person, this has to be transferred into the employee's passport. Some nurses I met had received their work permit document, but the transfer of their work permit to their passports was still refused by the Home Office. These nurses could not understand nor explain why these had been rejected. Some suspected that they were the victims of random Home Office checks or harassment.

At the time of my initial fieldwork, many accounts revealed that it was not only nurses who were unaware of the system, but that nursing home managers were ignorant too of the correct work permit process. Witness the case of Kiran who, on receipt of her NMC PIN, started looking for a full-time permanent job in England. She applied for many nursing jobs, and was offered one interview in a private nursing home in Wales. She attended the interview and was told she had been successful. She was delighted, as she desperately needed this job to live and work in the UK. When her employers tried to fast track a work permit for her however, the Home Office refused it, on the grounds that the employer had not followed the correct procedure when offering the post. Kiran felt that her failure to secure this post was due to the employer's lack of knowledge of the guidelines for employing a nurse from outside the EU.[12]

Guidelines for recruiting and employing health workers from countries outside of the EU are monitored, and all procedures are examined when the UK Home Office issues a work permit visa, but nurses felt these were not strictly followed. Once an institution obtains a work permit, the foreign employee then has to go to the Home Office, with the work permit document, to have a work permit visa issued. If a nurse changes her employment later, she has to obtain a new work permit for her new post. Kiran observed that, because of the complicated bureaucratic process, private sector employers were becoming increasingly hesitant about employing nurses from outwith the EU.

Because of these many hurdles, even after completing their adaptation training and obtaining an NMC PIN, for some nurses finding a full-time nursing job had not been easy. Nurses who had already obtained their NMC PIN had found themselves working only part-time in nursing homes, as bank nurses, for months and even years. It is hard to understand why these nurses could not find a job, while the RCN UK study report, at that time, was suggesting that Britain needed many more qualified nurses, and that hospitals and nursing homes were chronically under-staffed (Buchan & Seccombe 2009). Usha, on one occasion, travelled to Scotland from the Southeast of England for a job interview, and shared her experience:[13]

> I have been to so many places, almost every major city in Britain. I went to Ireland, Wales, and many places in England for job interviews. I have done my adaptation training and have obtained my PIN. But, finding a job is difficult. I asked for feedback after my interviews, they say that I did well and it was good, but I just don't get a job offer. My suspicion is when they learn that I need not just a job but a work permit as well, they just say sorry … I have over 20 years of working experience in Nepal. Presently I have a student visa, which allows me to work only 20 hours a week, but I need to work more than this in order to survive in this country. I don't understand why I don't get a full time RGN post.

In March 2009, Usha secured a full-time RGN post in a rural nursing home in Scotland. After obtaining her NMC PIN, it took her over a year to find a full-time nursing post with a work permit. She wanted to invite her children and husband, still in Nepal, to join her, but could not do so until she had a full-time job with a work permit. Around that time there were many others in the same situation, many of whom eventually found nursing home jobs, but only with much difficulty.

Even before the Home Office regulations changed, work permit policy was not clear to many nurses. In a 2008 interview of a Nepali nurse working in Scotland, she informed me that, when making work permit enquiries from Nepal, before coming to the UK, she was told that it would cost her an extra £1,000, on top of other agency fees. She thought it was a genuine official fee, so she paid this amount and obtained a work permit to work in a nursing home in England. But she could not explain the whole process any further, as she did not understand much about the regulation process herself. Another nurse in Scotland stated that she had a choice of a work permit or a student visa while she was in Nepal and preparing to come to the UK in 2004. An agent told her that the work permit costs were about £6,000 in total, inclusive of finding a job and adaptation placement in a nursing home, but that the adaptation student visa would cost only £3,500.

I interviewed Sheila, a UK returnee nurse in Kathmandu in autumn 2008, and she informed me that, despite going through the correct recruitment process, she was refused the transfer of her work permit visa to her passport. She shared her painful experience this way:[14]

> I went to Kemnay, in Aberdeenshire in October 2006. My visa was valid only until December 2006. So, I was under pressure to renew it and get an appropriate work permit. Soon after I started working in this nursing home, the nursing home manager started the work permit process, she sent some forms to the Home Office, but it took a long time to get any response. I made several enquiries, and finally I learnt that the form the manager had sent to the Home Office was not the right one, and it was for EU nationals only. Also, the nursing home manager, called Ms S., had a difficult working relation with the nursing home owner. And I sensed that the manager was much stressed; still she did reassure me that she would do the correct form soon. A month went by and nothing happened. Later Ms S. was sacked from the job, and then all the work permit process got stopped. There was a regional manager called Ms M. who came to work there. After Ms M. joined the team, I asked her to help me with the work permit and Ms M. sent new sets of paperwork to the Home Office for me. By this time, I did not have any valid visa; all the documents were already sent to the Home Office, waiting for a decision from the Home Office. I made further enquiries, phoned the Home Office again, and learnt that there were a couple more documents that were missing. They gave me two weeks to send all the missing but required papers. Later the Home Office suggested I go back to Nepal and apply for 'out-country work permit'. It was very stressful and disappointing, but I wanted to do it all correctly, so I left Scotland straight away. After I arrived in Kathmandu, I received further documents needed for the work permit from Ms M. and I made the work permit application here, but it was refused again. I know many nurses, some of my own friends who were in exactly similar positions; they did not have to go through the same process and the stress. So, how the Home Office makes decisions is not clear.

Another nurse working in Scotland in a nursing home in Lothian region said:[15]

> I sent my passport and all relevant documents for the work permit visa. I did not hear from the Home Office for months, and I got very stressed and worried. A friend suggested to me to contact a solicitor and I did that. He dealt with my application and my visa was approved.

She commented that, from her personal experience, this inconsistent British immigration policy has created business opportunities for private recruitment

agencies as well as immigration lawyers. Some of her friends have had problems in obtaining the right type of work permit visa, as their employers did
not fully know the procedure and the Home Office regulations.

Kiran, whom I introduced above as successful in her job interview in Wales
only for the Home Office to refuse her a work permit, was eventually offered
another job but had to leave her nursing home post after a month when her
passport came back from the Home Office with their refusal for the work
permit to be transferred into her passport. She was advised to go back to
Nepal to apply for her visa from there. Another Nepali nurse working in
Scotland related a very similar experience. Because of their fear that their
work permit would be refused by the Home Office, some nurses had been
extending their student visas just to remain in the country for a few more
years. At the time they had already obtained their NMC PIN, and were eligible to work as nurses, but they were working part-time casual shifts here
and there, despite being desperate for full-time nursing posts. Nurses, however, seemed determined that they were here to stay and to shape their
futures, and that they would do so by whatever means they could. Most
nurses believed that the Department of Health England's Code of Conduct
and the Home Office work permit policy were the main barriers to their
finding nursing jobs in the UK.

Department of Health Code of Practice for the International Recruitment of Healthcare Professionals (2004)

In the late 1990s, as many nurses from low-income countries started coming
to the UK, the inflow of nurses to Britain started to rise. Initially, South
Africa was losing its nurses to the UK at a time when the country itself was
experiencing an acute nursing shortage. Nelson Mandela, on his visit to
Britain in the early days of the Labour government in 1997, asked the British
Government not to recruit nurses from South Africa. He used his charisma
and political leverage to ensure Britain stopped nurse recruitment from his
country, utilising a humanitarian argument (Kingma 2006: 126–127). In 1999,
the Department of Health (DoH) in England produced a set of guidelines
that prohibited the NHS from recruiting nurses from South Africa. These
guidelines were further expanded in 2001 to include the Caribbean countries.
In 2003, a longer list of developing countries was added, at which time Nepal
was placed on the list. Finally in 2004, the guidelines were yet further
expanded to cover other categories of health workers, not just nurses.[16]
Although the DoH in England, where 90 per cent of internationally recruited
nurses were working at the time, developed the guidelines they were intended
for the National Health Services of all four UK countries.

Unfortunately, the Department of Health guidelines have no formal legal
basis. They are not mandatory rules that British employers are obliged to
implement. While the document bans active recruitment of nurses from
low-income countries such as Nepal, it says that, if a nurse from one of the

banned counties seeks employment in the UK independently, this is not restricted, at least in theory. Additionally, although clearly stated as intended for application by NHS trusts, the fast-growing private sector is not covered. These guidelines have also been criticised, as it is argued that they have no real effect on nurses coming to work in the UK from the very countries from where recruitment is banned, because of 'back door' recruitment (Buchan et al. 2005).

Nurses from the banned list of countries would come to the UK and work in the private sector for a while, then gradually filter into the NHS. This ban has actively diverted foreign nurses to the private sector, where the DoH guidelines were not followed, and where chances for a work permit visa for foreign nurses were higher, at least until 2006. It appears that the very policy intended to make the NHS an ethical employer, almost certainly has had 'unethical' consequences, as it has created a wider space for international recruitment agencies to link up with private nursing homes in the UK, where foreign nurses have been regularly exploited. Neither the DoH, nor the NMC, or any other authority appeared to have much control over this.

Adaptation to ever-changing and new visa regulations

In Chapter 2, we saw that not all nurses choose professional routes. Some come to the UK as dependent wives or as higher education students, depending on whichever visa appeared easiest for them to obtain. Two nurses might have come through two different channels with two different types of entry visa, but they usually have similar intentions: to work as nurses. Because of their visa status they can have quite different settling-in experiences. In general, nurses who have used IEC agents and have arrived in the UK as adaptation students, without a work permit, or as NVQ students, seem to get the worst deal. Many nurses who fall into this category have gone through a comparatively much more difficult time than those with work permits, or those who arrived as dependent wives or as higher education students.

The story presented earlier of the two young Nepali men on student visas, who went home from Scotland to marry, having asked their families to find them a 'nurse bride', is, as we noted, not an uncommon one (Shakya 2009; Ghimire 2007). A year later in January 2009 this number had increased and there were seven or eight Nepali nurses living and working in Scotland on dependent wives' visas, while their husbands were studying for university degrees. Nurses who joined their husbands in the UK tend to be fully supported, at least initially, during their early settling-in period. As these nurses held dependent visas, they had wider job options, and they could even work in the NHS, and most importantly their employers would not need to obtain work permits for them.

Those who came to study for master's degrees or other further education programmes, enrolled on their courses straight away, so they also had quite different arrival experiences. I interviewed only one nurse who came to study for an M.Sc. but who stayed longer. However, several informants stated that many nurses came to the UK for further studies. For this set of nurses, the transition experience must have been very different from that of those who came to the UK directly to work as nurses. The nurse I interviewed had a full scholarship for her master's degree, with all accommodation arrangements already made. After arrival she started her first university term, and so had plenty of time to go through the NMC PIN and job-seeking processes. She also had less financial pressure because she had a grant for her course.

Support and facilitation networks in the UK

After nurses arrive, existing support and facilitation networks in the UK play a vital role in their professional and social assimilation processes. Friends and family, migration agents and recently developed professional links have been the main support networks and social capital for newly arrived nurses. Those without personal access to professional links and family members in the UK, seemed to have relied on IEC agents for assistance in finding accommodation and jobs, and then helping them deal with work permit issues. Their settling-in experiences were, perforce, different from those with close family or other support networks. Many who had relied heavily on IEC agents and paid large fees found that, despite this, their job or adaptation placements were arranged only after they arrived here. For these nurses it had taken a longer time to settle. Those who had access to professional links, for example those who came to East Sussex with pre-planned adaptation courses, had their visa and work permits arranged by their employer. Some nurses have used multiple facilitation networks: migration agents as well as social support networks.

Professional links

I consider the link between Innovative Forum (introduced in Chapter 1) in Kathmandu and a private nursing home in East Sussex, England as an example of a 'professional link'. A few senior nurses had set up the Innovative Forum in Kathmandu to facilitate nurses' migration from Nepal to the UK. Given that the capacity of this network was small, only a few nurses have had access to this, but those who have used this link had direct contact with their future employer and their adaptation training facilitators. Everything required for a new nurse to settle in Britain was organised by a Nepal-educated nurse who had been working and living in East Sussex for many years. In total, this nursing home in East Sussex supported 78 Nepali nurses to have adaptation training and receive their NMC PIN. Some of the nurses came via the Innovative Forum, and others contacted the nursing home owner directly, with a small number contacting the home from other countries in which they were working.[17] Those with access to this link had a much smoother and easier transition. Namrata's story is a good example of this, and her arrival and survival experience has been very positive. She stated:[18]

I arrived here on the first of July 2005. I was picked up by a taxi from the airport. And there was really a good welcome from Nepali nurses – *Didi-Bahini* [older and younger sisters] who were already here. There was a hostel facility and I stayed there. Rosa Madam helped me to register for a National Insurance Number and to get all official documents ready. My accommodation [in East Sussex] was all arranged, Rosa Madam gave me a day to rest. I started working and adaptation training the day after I arrived. I shared a house with a few other Nepali nurses. They had organised a welcome programme for me, and I felt very comfortable and welcomed. I spent a full five months for the adaptation training and two weeks after I officially completed the training I received my NMC PIN. I paid a total of £1,000 fee for the adaptation course.

Another Nepali nurse came to the UK after working in Brunei for several years. Conducting all her communication with her future employer from Brunei, she managed to secure an adaptation placement in East Sussex. She said:[19]

I contacted Rosa Madam from Brunei while I was working there. As I felt I was a little familiar with nursing outside Nepal, I kind of expected what it would be like. I seemed fairly qualified and with plenty of work experience in Nepal and outside Nepal; they gave me a place to do an adaptation. I came here and went straight to East Sussex. I had no problem. I started the adaptation training a few days after I arrived. It took me a full three months to achieve what a qualified nurse is supposed to achieve, but I was in East Sussex for five months in total. It took me a while to get the NMC PIN. After I received my PIN, I applied for a job in London. It has been fairly smooth. I got this job in a private nursing-home in London and I am working there now as a qualified nurse.

Other nurses who came directly from Nepal also reported that, when they arrived in East Sussex, they were provided with accommodation, usually in a house with a few other Nepali nurses. This professional link seems to have been the cheapest and the most straightforward way to come to the UK, but had only limited capacity.

Facilitation or exploitation by IEC agents

Eva travelled to the UK with her friends, leaving her two young children and husband back in Nepal. After arriving in London she had hoped to under-take adaptation training, obtain her NMC PIN, and then find a nursing job as soon as possible.

When Eva was preparing to travel to the UK, she had applied for an adaptation student visa in 2005 in Kathmandu but it was refused. On decid-ing to try again, she was advised by an agent that she would not get a work permit visa or adaptation student visa, and was informed, falsely, that British visa regulations had changed in 2004. Following the agent's advice, she applied for, and obtained, an NVQ level 3 student visa on her second attempt. Her main intention, however, was to undertake adaptation training, not NVQ level 3 training, and this she was willing to do anywhere, in the NHS or privately, and as quickly as possible. She hoped to settle quickly and invite her husband and children over soon afterwards. When I met her in London, she was undertaking the ONP. She shared her early arrival and initial adjustment experiences:[20]

> Yes, we [herself and her two friends] arrived here on the 15th of September 2006; we arrived here early in the morning, somebody had come to meet us at the airport. The agent in Kathmandu had told us that they would put us in a hostel. We were prepared for that. From Heathrow, we went to Neasden in London, we were taken there by an agent, but when we arrived there, it was not a hostel. The house we were taken to was very small and very dirty and very congested. I was with two other friends; they did not like to stay there either, because it was very dirty and congested for them too. There were a few Nepali already in that house, one nurse *Bahini* (younger sister) and others who also had just arrived the night before, and someone else there. We found somewhere to put our bags down in their room. There was only one room, we refused to stay there and accept that room for three of us. The agents took us somewhere behind Neasden looking for other accommodation. We found a room, it was again fairly small, but with an attached kitchen and toilet but they wanted to put three people in one room and charge £65 a week per person. We did not want to pay so much, so we came back to the first place. It was getting late, we had nowhere else to stay that night, so we had to stay there with our Nepali nurse *Bahini*. We spent a night there ... although the agent did not want us to stay there [in somebody else's room], we just had to adjust in their one room, no choice. Next day we went to Aldershot to look for our friends. We stayed with friends in turns, one night with one friend and moved the next night to some other friends and some relatives, but we could not do that for long. We then found a place in Southall and moved here. Our friends helped us to find a room in Southall; my brother-in-law (*Jwain*) helped us to find a place. So we moved here. It took us about two weeks just to find somewhere to stay.

Sara had secured an adaptation student visa and had paid her IEC agent £5,000 in Nepal, all up front, for finding accommodation for her as well as an adaptation placement after her arrival in the UK. Having relied totally on an agent, her early experience was very unsettling. When I met her in a small village, near Bicester in Buckinghamshire in 2007, she had lived in various parts of Britain over the previous year, going through many difficulties, and finally was under adaptation training in a nursing home there. The IEC agent arranged her initial accommodation in London, but it was also very cramped and in poor condition, and she felt cheated. As she phrased it:[21]

> It seemed OK initially, but trouble started once we went back to London. Mr Sam [the agent] had not arranged any accommodation for us but we were told that everything would be done for us. We were taken to an Indian's house. We were kept in a waiting-room, in a very strange house. The landlord did not have any room to rent out, but Mr Sam kept us in a waiting-room, while he went to negotiate with the landlord privately in a different room. Later they gave us a room with a single bed for two of us to share. The room was very *transparent, glass* window with no *curtain*. Many males were living in that house in small rooms and no *curtain*, just two of us female. We were very scared. It was terrible, just so bad.

A few days after her arrival, her agent sent Sara to Northern Ireland with some other Nepali nurses, for an initial three months of English language training. About five weeks later, Sara and other nurses were asked to return to London, the reason given for this being that the language course fee was too expensive. The agent also told her that no adaptation training was available in Northern Ireland, and he was trying hard to arrange a placement for them in London. Sara and her friends came back to London. Once again there was no proper accommodation arranged for them when they arrived. They had to share a room in a house, but were assured this was only temporary. She said she: 'could not believe that people in London lived like that, in such poor conditions'. As there was no adaptation training arranged for them, this temporary measure was extended for many weeks, with no jobs. The money they had brought with them from home was about to run out, and the future seemed very uncertain. She was extremely stressed; she stated: 'How can one live like that with so much stress, no job, no money and no support? I nearly *cracked* ...'

Kripa used an agent in Kathmandu to first help her obtain a UK visa, and then expected this agent to find her a nursing post after arrival here. She had applied for a visa to do NVQ level 3, as per advice from an agent in Kathmandu. She was told that this course would take between eight and 12 months. She was given an 18-month student visa. The agent had also told her that somebody would pick her up from Heathrow Airport and take her to pre-booked accommodation in London. Before she left Nepal she paid the agent £370 as a month's rent, and another £50 for somebody to take her to the accommodation. She said that she had arrived at Heathrow at around 7 a.m. with Gulf Air, but there was nobody there to meet her. She had no choice, she said, but to wait, hoping that somebody would come and take her to her new accommodation. But no one came. Eventually she rang the contact person in London, but had difficulty even making this first phone call. She stated:[22]

Everything was completely alien to me. To begin with I did not have the right kind of money, but managed to get some change. I put the coins in the phone box, then something happened with the phone, and needed more coins. I could not even contact the person I wanted to contact, and did not get the coins back either. Then I had to go upstairs to find somebody at the help desk. Finally I managed to contact another agent in London but he told me that it was Sunday, and that he would not even send me a taxi and, with no accommodation ready for me, I should stay with a friend for a few days. I was very stressed-out.

Fortunately I had a friend's contact number, so I rang her. This friend sent me a taxi to the airport to take me to her place in East London. I arrived there by two in the afternoon. I stayed there for a few days, but I had to move out, as there was not enough room for so many people already there. Later I contacted the agent again. The accommodation they arranged for me was very expensive. Another friend of mine was living in the Wembley area. I went and stayed there for about two weeks. While I was there, I started looking for a job or adaptation placement, or anything. Luckily, I found this place in East Sussex, I spoke with the matron of this nursing home, and the matron said that she could put me on a waiting list for adaptation, but in the meantime I could start working as a carer. I lost a month's rent that I had paid to the agent in Kathmandu. I got nothing back, not even a cup of tea.

It was only after almost a month of unsettlement in London, moving from one friend's place to another, continuously searching for an adaptation placement, that Kripa travelled to East Sussex for an interview. She said:

When I went to East Sussex for an interview, I had also applied for CRB checks and was told that the process may take up to two months. I prepared myself to wait for the CRB report. A few days later, I was contacted by the Matron. If I wanted to start working I could do so, but starting with a few hours a week. I was delighted that I got something; initially I worked for about four hours a day and some weeks only eight hours a week in total, like this. Fortunately, there became a space available for me to start adaptation early, and I completed adaptation in February.

According to the employment regulations in place at the time in the UK, anybody who worked with the elderly, children and vulnerable people needed to be checked by the Criminal Record Bureau (CRB) and their record should be clean.[23] It appears that not all employers follow these government regulations. Before starting working in private nursing homes, some nurses had CRB checks and some did not. Nurses mentioned further inconsistencies with employment regulations. Some were asked to wait for CRB clearance first, after their arrival in the UK, but this does not seem to have been the case with all nurses I met. At the time, the CRB check normally took between four and six weeks. It was not clear when and why some nurses needed CRB clearance and others did not before starting work. One explanation might be that CRB clearance, prior to starting work, seems to depend on how urgently a nurse's services are needed by her employer. Nurses I interviewed had very little understanding of the employment regulations and UK government policy on working hours and working terms and conditions. Kripa's experience illustrates how private sector employers manipulate the system.

As highlighted previously, the number of internationally qualified nurses waiting for adaptation training placements started to rise, and finding placements became difficult, even for agents. Nurses became more proactive, as revealed by Hema, whom I met in East Sussex. She had arrived in Britain in 2004, and told me that after their arrival, she and a few friends decided to rent a room in London, right next to where their agent lived. This was deliberately done in order to see the agent, and nag him every day to help them find adaptation training placements.

News and rumours circulate fast, so some nurses who came to the UK via an agency with an NVQ student visa learned quickly that nurses in East Sussex had better luck than some others in London. Accordingly some of them moved to East Sussex within a few days of their arrival in London, despite making no prior arrangements with the private nursing home. They felt that East Sussex had a bigger Nepali community and a better support network, through which they imagined it would be easier for them to achieve their goals. Several of the nurses I met chose this route.

Moti had used an agent to obtain an NVQ student visa to come to the UK in 2006, and later went to East Sussex in search of an adaptation placement. She came to England on her own, leaving her husband behind in Nepal. When I met her in East Sussex in March 2008, her husband had arrived just a few weeks before from Nepal and was still trying finding his way around. I was invited to join them for lunch in their flat. Moti had just returned from her night shift in a nursing home. Although she looked very tired, she wanted to stay up and talk before she went to bed. We cooked together and chatted. Over our meal she shared her experiences of becoming a nurse, of arriving and surviving in Britain. She said:[24]

> After I landed here, the first difficulty was to find a place to stay, and sort out the adaptation training. Finding a place for adaptation has been the hardest of all, but life has not been easy even after I received NMC PIN. With so much stress I completed the adaptation training and received my PIN. Then my next challenge came, I started looking for a full-time RGN post. But this has been very difficult. It is like ... I go through one set of troubles, feel a bit happier and start seeing a light towards the end of a long tunnel but that disappears quickly, and another set of problems arrive.

First problem was I could not find a place to be an adaptation student. I was already here as a [NVQ level 3] student. Then there was the change of NMC and ONP policy [regarding registration for overseas trained nurses] and I got caught by it; it got more difficult for us. Before, many nurses did not need an IELTS, now we need to obtain 7 score, it is very difficult to get. I struggled through that, worked hard and got the required score, then I had to face the entire problem with adaptation and PIN; I struggled through this again, told myself to be brave, worked through the difficult times and got my PIN. Now getting a job has become another hurdle. I went to so many interviews in all four countries in the UK; every time I was told that I did well in the interview but never got a job. I have got my PIN, it has been almost a year now, and I still have to work as a carer. I have no idea why I don't get a job, but now people are very reluctant to offer a job to a foreigner who needs a work permit. Last time I went to Scotland for a job interview. I was offered a job in a nursing home in rural Scotland; they have a new nursing home just recently opened. I have been told that I can start working there whenever I am ready. I have resigned from my job here in East Sussex and am hoping to move to Scotland soon, but let's wait and see. I would not be surprised if more troubles come ahead. It feels like I live in East Sussex, I just go over one set of difficulties, and feel low and recover again, then the next set of difficulties arise.

I live in East Sussex now, but I feel that there are more troubles coming towards me from London. There is no end to this chain of troubles. I have been here for almost two years. How long can I stay like this? It feels like *Kahilai Nasasakine Samashyaharuko Sikri* [a never ending chain of difficulties]. Troubles come one after another.

A few months later Moti and her husband moved to Scotland from East Sussex, taking all their belongings with them. She began work in a nursing home in a small village on the east coast, whilst her husband started looking for a job or any further educational opportunity. I was in regular contact with them. Moti's new manager had applied for a work permit for her, which arrived in time. Later all the paperwork was forwarded to the Home Office, for transfer of the work permit to her passport, and for the new dependant's visa for her husband. She was working and waiting for the passport to come back from the Home Office. When their passports were returned, they realised that the work permit visa had not been granted. By then their old visas had expired. She had the job and work permit, but why the Home Office had refused to give her a work permit visa was not clear to them, and there was no explanation proffered. They travelled down to the Home Office, in Croydon, London, the very next day to find out in person what had happened. There they were advised to go back to Nepal and submit their application from there. They were very stressed and disheartened.

Just before they left for Nepal, in early summer, 2008, Moti phoned me:[25]

> It has been a full two years I have been going through these types of
> tensions and stresses. We have gone through so much; waste of money
> and, time and so much mental torture to bear with it. After all this, now
> we have to go back home.

Once back in Nepal they both felt extremely anxious and stressed about the
whole process of changing their visa status. Their reapplication for a work
permit for the UK cost them another two months of stress, and a seemingly
endless wait. Their future seemed very uncertain. Finally a work permit was
granted and they returned to Scotland in August of that year. It had indeed
been an endless chain of troubles for them.

For a few other nurses, the whole migration experience has been very
negative. A UK returnee nurse told me her story in Kathmandu in autumn
2008:[26]

> When I arrived in London early in the morning by night flight, I was met
> at the airport by my *Jwain* [brother-in-law]. I went with him to Lewi-
> sham, where he lived. He shared a three bedroom flat with three other
> Nepali families. He had a room, and a shared kitchen and toilet/bath-
> room. It was a shock for me, I asked myself, was I really in London? A
> few days after I arrived, I contacted the Real Dream agent in London as
> I was facilitated by them in Kathmandu and had paid all agency fees up
> front. I was told that I would get something soon. A week went by and
> nothing happened. I contacted them again and I was reassured regularly
> that they were trying their best; all would happen soon, I would get a
> placement for adaptation course. I was waiting for this. My *Jwain* was
> busy, working in a restaurant part-time and was a student as well. He did
> not have any time for me and there was nobody else to take me and show
> me around. I got used to spending days watching television and feeling
> restless. Every time I contacted the agents I would get the same reassur-
> ance from them. One month went by but nothing happened. I could no
> longer stay like that. I moved to Burnt Oak, to stay with my husband's
> friend. From there, too, I contacted the agent regularly, but received the
> same old message. I met some other Nepali nurses in London, many of
> them were in the same situation, and I learnt that the documents I was
> given by the agents in Kathmandu about adaptation course at *Tudor
> College*, and placement at *Elizabeth Hospital* were all *fraud*. Some of the
> nurses in London phoned Tudor College and Elizabeth Hospital but
> learnt that they were enrolled neither for any course nor for clinical pla-
> cement for adaptation training. The agent said that they should not do
> the pre-adaptation course because it was going to be very expensive but
> that they would get the adaptation course straight. I and some other
> nurses I met in London felt confused with this information, as we had

visas to do the pre-adaptation course. Yet, the agent insisted that they did not try it, because it would be too expensive, and if we really wanted to do it we would need to pay for it ourselves. But we thought that we had already paid for this in Nepal, that 5 lakh rupees [approximately £4,000–4,500] covered it all. Another four to five months went by, nothing happened, I was missing my family in Nepal. No job, no adaptation there and I continued to stay with my friends for five more months in Burnt Oak, until February 2006.

Her difficulties in fact continued for some time. She lived in Britain for almost 20 months. During that time she never felt settled, as she did not have a secure job. The inappropriate visa gave her no sense of security. She finally returned to Nepal in March 2007.

From the NMC UK record of 527 fully licensed Nepali nurses in the UK, only 78 had access to appropriate professional links, and had experienced relatively smoother settling-in experiences. The majority of nurses have faced many challenges with personal and professional assimilation, and have ended up working in private nursing homes. Despite their trials, nurses said their desire was ultimately to work in the NHS, even though this was currently not possible, due to the 'ethical' recruitment policy and nurses' visa status.

Conclusion

This chapter has shown that, since the year 2000, Nepali nurses' international migration had been increasing, with the flow to the UK seeming to have increased in 2005–2006, and levelling off thereafter until the global economic crisis and UK policy changes in the regulation of international recruitment made life so very much more difficult.

How quickly and smoothly migrant nurses have undergone their transition has been determined by when they migrated and the types of entry routes and visas chosen, and crucially their access to support networks in the UK. Those who arrived before 2004, when the DoH strengthened its guidelines for ethical recruitment of overseas healthcare professionals, had easier transitions than those who arrived subsequently. But other factors, such as social and professional networks, have been equally important. Those who had professional links with the Innovative Forum and with a private nursing home in East Sussex, for example, were better received and supported throughout the process until they obtained their work permits. Those who arrived after 2004 relied increasingly on the proliferating number of IEC agents and had the worst times at every stage in their initial settling-in process. A very small number of wives, who received a dependant's visa, had a relatively easier transition.

Despite a greater need for more qualified nurses in Britain's NHS, there is no easy way for Nepali nurses to secure NHS jobs. Arriving in the UK, and struggling with regulations, jobs and visas, has been tough for the majority of nurses. Smith et al. (2006) found that, in the context of international nurses' migration, those who were recruited by the NHS, and entered into the NHS in groups, have better arrival and settling-in experiences. In 2000–2001, overseas nurses, recruited directly by employers had their work permit visas, adaptation programmes, accommodation facilities and other administrative procedures handled by those employers, who even organised a 'meet-and-greet' programme, where nurses were given a start-up pack of food and telephone cards (RCN 2003). Unfortunately, Nepali nurses have not been members of such comparatively privileged groups, and there has been no such organised official nurse recruitment from Nepal.

We have also seen that the DoH Code of Practice on International Recruitment of Healthcare Professionals, which was developed to promote ethical practices, has failed. Instead it has created the space for the poorly regulated private sector to exploit foreign migrant nurses. These ethical guidelines are supposed to help low-income countries like Nepal to retain their valuable resources. Yet it has been quite evident that, in Nepal, it has made no difference, as the country continues to be a prominent nurse-supplying country to the global nursing labour market.

In Chapter 1, we saw how women in Nepal are dependent on family and close support networks. When they arrive in the UK this support is absent, and they are highly vulnerable and prone to exploitation. A new culture of living and working has to be adjusted to rapidly. We have seen how migrant nurses have gone through and experienced the initial hurdles: the lack of support from their mentors during their adaptation training; the poor standard of training guidelines; and the inconsistencies with employment policies, such as CRB checks. Despite such difficulties, apart from a very few who returned to Nepal, most nurses have made adjustments and adapted to their new professional and social lives. The next chapter will explore their working lives in detail, and their reflections on career successes and achievements during their time in the UK.

Notes

1 This is a Nepali nurses' diaspora organisation in the UK, and is further discussed in Chapter 5.
2 Email communication with Public Relations Officer, NMC UK, June 2007 and with Customer Information and Data Request Officer, Quality Improvement Team, June 2019.
3 I received this information from the British Embassy in Kathmandu in 2007. The NVQ levels 3 and 4 are not run by the NMC, but are run by many private colleges. They do not lead to registration with the NMC, which would allow the holder to work in nursing in the UK, and do not have an IELTS – an International English Language Testing System – requirement as one of their entry criteria. Those who successfully complete an NVQ level 4 course usually end up working as carers, as the course does not qualify them to work as nurses. But the ONP is approved by the NMC. Successful completion of this course leads to an NMC PIN, which allows the holder to work in nursing sector in the UK. Email communication with the Consul in the British Embassy, Kathmandu, December 2006.

4 Entry criteria for ONP were that: (a) an internationally qualified nurse should have a valid NMC decision letter; (b) he/she should have an IELTS score of 7 in all categories (many Nepali nurses find it very hard to obtain the required IELTS score); and (c) if already living and working in the UK the nurse will receive priority.

5 Work permits were, however, tied to a workplace where employees were to stay for four years. If they changed their jobs, their work permits would become invalid, and they would need new ones to work in a different place.

6 www.nmc.org.uk/globalassets/sitedocuments/registration/registering-nurse-or-midwife-outside-eu.pdf, accessed on 2/5/2019.

7 Interviewed in Edinburgh, Scotland, June 2006.

8 Email communication with the Publicity Officer of NMC, May 2008. How this number came down to 193 from over 37,000 is not clear. One possible reason could be that many internationally educated nurses gave up attempting NMC registration or were just removed from the NMC list, as their prescribed period for adaptation/ONP training expired.

9 Due in the most part to these changes, gradually Nepali nurses stopped coming to the UK and, within a decade, the number in 2018 has again become almost insignificant.

10 Except one who found an NHS adaptation placement, as she came here as a dependent spouse so she did not require an adaptation student visa or work permit.

11 Interviewed in Aberdeen, Scotland, January 2008.

12 The policy is as follows: when there is a vacancy, the employer has to advertise locally first, then nationally, and wait for a month. By the end of this time, if there is no local or national applicant available, then they can offer the position to an international candidate. They need to submit all the evidence of efforts made to recruit local/national candidates, for example job advertisements, to the Home Office with a correct application for work permit for their new employee. Then the Home Office, in theory, would issue a work permit. Finally, the nurse has to send her passport, work permit and employment contract to the Home Office for a work permit to be placed in her passport.

13 Interviewed in East Sussex, England, April 2008.

14 Interviewed in Kathmandu, Nepal, October 2008.

15 Interviewed Edinburgh, Scotland, June 2008.

16 In fact, the DoH England prided itself for being the first country in the world to develop ethical guidelines for international recruitment of nurses and health workers (DoH 2004).

17 I met and interviewed four nurses who had come to do their adaptation in East Sussex. Three of them used the Innovative Forum in Nepal and one came directly from Brunei.

18 Interviewed in East Sussex, England, February 2008.

19 Interviewed in London, England, March 2007.

20 Interviewed in London, England, April 2008.

21 Interviewed in Buckinghamshire, England, February 2007.

22 Interviewed in London, England, March 2008.

23 CRB clearance is a police check. Applicants' criminal records are checked by police and reported to the employer, and a copy is sent to the applicant.

24 Interviewed in East Sussex, England, March 2008.

25 Telephone conversation, April 2008.

26 Interviewed in Kathmandu, Nepal, October 2008.

4 'There is a vast difference from what I had thought'

Professional life in the UK

In the last chapter, I discussed Nepali nurses' experience of their arrival and initial settling in the UK, focussing mainly on their struggle to obtain the all-important NMC PIN, and then nursing jobs with work permit visas. In this chapter I continue to explore their professional lives. I discuss the nature of nursing work, working conditions and workload, and nurses' relationships with their patients, patients' relatives, colleagues and line managers. Sumi's story is a good place to begin, as it encompasses all these issues.

Sumi's experience: a case study

I met Sumi for the first time in Scotland in the summer of 2007 and I have remained in touch with her regularly until today. She was then a young, single woman perhaps in her mid-20s, dynamic and talented. She came to the UK in December 2004, with a dream of becoming a Cardiac Care Nurse in a Cardiac Care Unit (CCU) in a high-tech hospital.

After graduating as a staff nurse in 2001, Sumi had applied for a CCU nursing post in Gangalal Heart Centre in Kathmandu, the country's most advanced heart care centre. Competition was so fierce that Sumi did not get the job. She was very disappointed but continued to aim for a CCU nursing post. Within a few months she was offered a staff nurse post in another of Kathmandu's private and modern teaching hospitals, working there first as a surgical nurse, before moving on to become a CCU and Intensive Care Unit (ICU) nurse. She also worked in other departments in rotation for over three years. One of the main reasons she wanted to come to Britain was to fulfil her dream of obtaining cardiac care experience in a technologically advanced healthcare system.

Sumi's interest in moving to Britain stemmed from the time that many of her social and professional colleagues were coming to the UK around 2003–2004. She too began to imagine living a successful life, with better professional opportunities in the UK. She met no major family resistance, nor had she any commitments that would have prevented her move. Indeed her parents, brothers and sisters fully supported her. She made all necessary preparations and arranged an adaptation placement through a friend, who was already working in the UK. With her friend's help she found a training place and paid £4,500 in total in adaptation training fees: £1,000 as a deposit in Nepal before making a visa application to travel to the UK, and the remaining £3,500 before she started her training. She felt fortunate to have a close friend already working in the UK to find her a training place without much difficulty, though it was costly. She managed to negotiate all the common hurdles, already explored in detail: the visa process in Nepal and the many initial challenges with adaptation placements and NMC registration in the UK. She finally received her NMC PIN in December 2005.

Sumi felt that working in the nursing home, where she did her adaptation training, was a completely 'multicultural' experience, for it was staffed almost exclusively by a migrant workforce from international sources. She worked with nurses from the Philippines, India and Pakistan, and the nursing home owner was from Pakistan and the manager was Sri Lankan. She commented that, at times, it did not feel as if she was in Britain. She found herself not professionally stimulated during this period, as nursing home work proved slow and very basic. With no new nursing skills to learn and practise, Sumi felt that she was actually deskilling herself, moving further and further away from CCU/ICU nursing. One year in a nursing home was long enough for her, during which time she lost her professional confidence, even to work as a general nurse in an acute hospital clinical setting, quite apart from her dreamed-for high-tech CCU or ICU job. She realised that there was no chance for her to learn any advanced nursing skills, let alone use any of the simple nursing procedures she was used to in her previous post in Nepal. She decided to look for a new job, one that would ideally lead her towards specialising in cardiac care nursing.

After receiving her NMC-PIN, she started looking for a full-time staff nurse post; preferably in CCU. She made some enquiries about CCU jobs but learnt that all CCU posts were attached to NHS hospitals, and she was not eligible for one. In desperation, she moved to Birmingham where she had a close friend, who was also a nurse from Nepal. She stayed with her friend there. While in Birmingham she continued to look for a job. She said:

> Here [in Scotland], my *Daju* [elder cousin brother] was here in the university. And I decided to leave there [East Sussex], but I did not know where to go and where to start from. I thought it would be better, and easier to be near somebody I know. My friend, who just phoned me [she had received a phone call during our interview], wanted me to go to Birmingham. I went there for a week. I did not look for work there, but I stayed in her place. I did not like the area very much. News [of Birmingham] was then very negative at that time, I heard about racial tension and fights. I did not apply for any job there. While I was there I asked my *Daju* to find me some contact telephone numbers of some nursing homes from the Yellow Pages. He gave me a few numbers, and then I rang some nursing homes. One nursing home said, 'Come and

work from tomorrow.' I said 'I am not in Scotland now, I am in Birmingham now, so I can't come tomorrow but I can come the day after tomorrow'. Next day, I booked my ticket to Scotland, and then started working the day after that. Forget about the interview, they did not even have time for any paperwork, no work permit, nothing. They were so desperate I started working the next day. And also, people here were not aware that nurses from overseas would require [a] work permit to work here. They took it like they were employing a British citizen; they employed me like I was a local person.

Sumi was disappointed not to have been able to work in a CCU, but she accepted the fact that she lacked choice and flexibility about what kind of job she wanted and where it might be. To gain that kind of opportunity, she found that she would need to wait for a further five years to qualify for 'Permanent Residency' status, and only then would she be allowed to enter the NHS. She prepared herself to wait for this, as there was no other quick and easy route to fulfil her dream. Forced to accept the circumstances, she decided to apply for any nursing home job, for at the time any job seemed better than no job. Although this nursing home was in a small village, it was within commutable distance from the city centre where she was living, and there were regular bus services, and she could live near her relatives. So, after a period of unsettling experiences in the Southeast of England, she finally moved to Scotland in the summer of 2006.

Sumi secured her first nursing home position very easily, without even a proper interview process, but she then faced the difficulty of sorting out her work permit. She knew little about work permit regulations and application processes, and her nursing home manager was not fully aware of these issues either. The process was delayed, but she had already started working there. She knew that she would need a work permit to work legally, but all this was in her manager's hands and she could do little about it, which compounded her stress levels.

After being there for a while she felt that the nursing home manager was not very supportive, was maybe racist, and certainly a bully. Sumi felt that she was being targeted and constantly harassed. It became unbearable and, as she was becoming increasingly stressed, she began to look for an alternative job. Some of her work colleagues were also bullies. She just felt lonely and vulnerable. At one stage she contacted the RCN, the nurses' trade union body, for help. An RCN representative visited her work place and spoke with the manager and other work colleagues:

Yes, she [manager] said she is a very good staff member and she is very reliable staff member, etc. What could the RCN representative say? Nothing! She [the manager] appeared very nice. Who would they believe, what could they say? They first said *RCN will not tolerate any racism at all, we will do some action* [in English] but when they visited they did not find any problem.

She continued, 'They [the manager and some of her colleagues] called me friend and in front of the RCN representative, they praised me for how hard I worked and for being a good team player and a good colleague, etc..'

It seemed as if there was nothing to investigate, so the RCN representative left with no further action. But the day after the representative's visit, everything went back to the way it was before. Sumi felt there was no point in staying there and that it would be better and healthier for her to be in a different place. The following conversation illustrates this:

SUMI: This is my feeling anyway. I felt that I was harassed.

RADHA: Can you give me some examples of how you were harassed? You mentioned you felt that you were picked on more than other staff ... anything else?

SUMI: For example, we all are working hard and we always have staff shortages, staffing is a common problem, in some shifts we were like supposed to have six staff but, only two come on duty, it could get this bad [staff present], and we [as a registered nurse and the shift in-charge] have to deal with everything.

RADHA: Why only two, because of people off sick or just no staff in the rota?

SUMI: Off sick, or they just report off sick. When you work under a stressful environment, of course you miss out some work, we all do. When some colleagues miss some work, it is OK. But when I miss out something, she [the manager] would pick on me, only me. Some colleagues noticed this too and they asked 'why is it always you that gets picked on?' It was like nit picking, I felt I was picked on excessively, so [she had just] decided to leave that place. This is the main reason [for leaving the work].

While working in the nursing home, she continued to hold on to her dream of returning to cardiac care nursing, but felt that she really had no real choice but to wait for another couple of years. Sometimes, she continued, 'it felt like too long to wait, and at other times so close to getting PR', and thus reaching her goal. While working in this nursing home, she thought she should at least learn a bit about NHS work and gain some experience in her own spare time. At one point she became very impatient, so just decided to do some NHS nurse-bank work in her days off.

Accordingly, she joined the NHS nurse-bank as a possible stepping-stone into the NHS and also to find out about the system. This was a viable option, as she now had a work permit for the nursing home, and with this permit was able to work part-time in the NHS. She had an induction day for bank nursing and started working one day a week, and in some weeks for just a few hours, during her days off. She said she was happy that she had started working in the NHS for the first time in the UK, but at the same time, she found it very hard to adjust to the new working environment. She found staff to be not very supportive. Some were even racist and she experienced harassment there too. The ward in which she worked was just another long-term elderly care unit. Work was thus very similar to her everyday nursing home work: not at all like working in CCU. She tried it for a few months, but reached a point of it being so emotionally draining, and yielding so little achievement, that she stopped. By this time she had spent over a year in Scotland.

Sumi still had a few years to wait for 'Permanent Residency' status. She felt however that she should not waste her time, but keep trying to find a stimulating job or a course. She began to look for a part-time university course that would perhaps direct her towards further CCU/ICU training and a job. Having made all relevant Internet searches, she found out there was an 'open day' in the university nearby, running nursing and health science courses, including Cardiac Care Nursing. She went there with much enthusiasm, met the Cardiac Care Nursing course organiser, and expressed her interest to enrol on the course. She learned, however, that all cardiac care training courses were attached to clinical posts, and were intended for those who were already working in the field, in NHS hospitals, as a part of a continuing professional development programme. She returned home with yet another disappointment.

Sumi's work in the nursing home had never been a satisfying experience, nor did it provide her with the work experience she sought. She also felt that she could not have any social life with the people at work, the same people who would make stereotyped racist comments at work, such as: 'How can you stay so slim and eat curry every day?' She spent most of her days off on the Internet, chatting with family and friends in Nepal, or visiting her Nepali friends and relatives in the town in which she lived, or watching DVD films. She eventually found a nursing job, in a different nursing home, very close to her rented flat in the city centre, and started working there. It was at this point I met her for the first time, interviewing her in the summer of 2007. I met with her several times, became part of her social network and I remain in touch. For several years after our initial meeting, she remained keen on a CCU position. She eventually received her 'Permanent Residency' and continued to look for a CCU nursing opportunity. In 2014, she was offered a Research Nurse post, and has been working with an NHS healthcare research team since then.

Many of the younger nurses I met had dreams like Sumi's, of furthering their professional careers, but until they have been granted 'Permanent Residency' status the majority have no professional choices. This is not only the experience of Nepali nurses either. Overseas nurses, coming to the UK from countries outside the EU, have to endure similar difficulties, as they try to obtain visas and work permits. Eventually they become not only deskilled, but also de-motivated about looking for career progression opportunities (Larsen 2007). A lack of choice in jobs, racial discrimination and bullying and harassment at work are all too common and are shared by many migrant nurses globally (Dicicco-Bloom 2004; Henry 2008). These issues are now examined in detail, starting with nurses' working conditions.

Nurses' working condition and working life

I charted the qualifications and the experiences of the nurses I interviewed. Table 4.1 illustrates Nepali migrant nurses' professional mobility. It looks first at their professional qualification in Nepal and where they were on a career ladder, and then at the point where they joined the professional career ladder on arrival in the UK, where they were professionally at the time of the research interviews in the UK, and a decade later in early 2019.

Type of nursing and workplace

The table above illustrates that the majority of Nepali nurses had had further education in Nepal after their initial staff nurse training; some even had master's level qualifications. However, when they arrived in the UK, all but one had to start their professional careers as carers in privately run nursing homes. For them the easiest entry point, or the only option available, was this kind of setting. The two nurses who did not need work permits because they had dependants' visas were working in NHS hospitals. Nurses related that their IEC agents in Nepal had reassured them that they would secure nursing home jobs easily. But the nurses' understanding of the nature of private nursing home work was based on their knowledge of nursing homes in Nepal, and so they travelled to the UK with false expectations.

Nursing home and care work: a culture shock

Almost all the nurses I interviewed confirmed that IEC agents in Nepal failed to properly explain the nature of the work involved, having reassured them it would be a straightforward process to obtain posts. There was little or no understanding about the nature of nursing work in the UK.[1] Nurses said that before coming to the UK they had neither seen, nor looked after, patients who were so dependent on carers and nursing staff for their healthcare and all their daily personal care needs, and on such a long-term basis. Many nurses, when exposed to nursing homes for the first time in the UK, experienced considerable work-related 'culture shock', as can be seen from the following accounts.

Kiran, whom I introduced in Chapter 2, came to Britain with over ten years of work experience and a BN degree in Hospital Nursing in Nepal. She arrived in the UK in July 2005. As previously briefly described, in Nepal she had worked in a 'British-style' healthcare system, run by the British authorities for Gurkha families. She revealed:[2]

> We used to get the *Nursing Standard, Nursing Times* and *Nursing Research* journals. I used to read through them every month to update on new research evidence in nursing. My main job there was to work as what would be equivalent to a Health Visitor here in Britain. I kept up all immunisation records, managed hypertension and diabetes, chronic

Table 4.1 Nurses' professional mobility before and after migration to the UK

Respondent	Qualification	Last nursing position in Nepal	First nursing position in UK	Position at the time of interview	Position in 2019 (ten years later)
01	SN, BN Med.	Programme manager in an INGO	Carer in a NH	Night nurse in a NH	SN in an NHS hospital in England
02	SN	ICU/CCU nurse	Carer in a NH	Carer in a NH	Part-time carer in an NHS hospital and dental nursing
03	SN, BN	SN in a government hospital	Carer	SN in a NH	SN in an NHS hospital in England
04	SN, BN	CCU nurse	Carer	Carer in a NH	SN in a care home in England
05	SN	School nurse	Carer	Carer in a NH	Not known
06	SN, BN, PG in Women's Studies and M.Ed.	Various INGOs management positions	Carer	SN in a NH	SN in an NHS hospital in England
07	SN, BN	Nurse lecturer, Reproductive Health Co-ordinator for a foreign aid funded project	Carer	SN in a NH	NHS hospital in England
08	SN, BN	Nurse lecturer	Carer	Carer/ONP student	SN in NHS hospital
09	SN, specialist CCU nurse	CCU/ICU nurse in a major teaching hospital in Kathmandu	Carer	SN (night) in a NH	SN in NHS Hospital
10	SN	Maternity nurse/midwife (government position)	Carer	SN in a NH	SN in a NH
11	SN	CCU/ICU and surgical nurse	Carer	SN in rural NH	M.Sc. graduate; research nurse

Respondent	Qualification	Last nursing position in Nepal	First nursing position in UK	Position at the time of interview	Position in 2019 (ten years later)
12	SN	Orthopaedic nurse	Carer	SN in NH	SN in NHS hospital
13	SN	Orthopaedic nurse	Carer	Carer in NHS hospital	Returned to Nepal
14	SN, BPH, M.Sc. in Public Health	Management position in an INGO	Carer- but came to Britain as an MSc student	SN in a NH	Ph.D. student
15	SN, BN, MPH	Management position in an INGO	Carer	SN in a NH	Ph.D. graduate, SN in various NHs
16	SN	OT/surgical nurse	Carer	SN in a NH	SN in an NHS hospital in England
17	SN, BN	Family health nurse	Carer	SN in a NH	SN in an NHS hospital in England
18	SN	Eye specialist Nurse	Carer	SN in an NHS eye clinic	SN in an NHS hospital eye clinic.
19	SN	Maternity nurse/midwife	Carer	Carer in a NH (but had NMC PIN)	SN in a NH
20	SN, specialist midwifery trained	Birthing centre nurse with specialist midwifery training	Carer	Carer in a NH (but had NMC PIN)	SN in an NHS hospital in England
21	SN, BN	O.T. nurse in a major teaching hospital in Kathmandu	Carer	SN (night) in a NH	SN in an NHS hospital in England

Source: Research fieldwork data

Note: ONP = Overseas Nurses Programme; NH = nursing home; SN = staff nurse or registered nurse wounds, etc. I thought that nursing in Britain would be like that and from what I read in the *Nursing Standard* that it would be more innovative and evidence-based. But when I first went to my very first nursing home, I was totally shocked, shocked by the fact that I saw very thin and mal-nourished elderly women, and in the same place, extremely overweight and totally dependent women. I had never seen or used any kind of hoists or moving aids to transfer totally dependent patients before I came here. I felt like crying, I did not know how I would be able to handle this, how I could work there. My expectations were 90 per cent wrong.

Another young, private school educated and private college trained nurse, Suruchi, who came to Britain in 2005 shared her experience:[3]

I went into nursing because I wanted to go abroad. From Nepal, it [nursing] seemed like the easiest route to get any opportunity abroad. I was trained in one of the private colleges in Pokhara, attached to a big modern private hospital under the management of the Manipal group. I was not sure about the nursing work in a practical sense, but I really liked teaching, and I wanted to be a nurse teacher. After I was qualified, I got a job with an NGO [non-governmental organisation]. My parents owned and ran an English boarding school and I worked there for a while as a school nurse. I then came to the UK to do NVQ level 4. My expectation of healthcare and nursing was that it would be very technologically advanced and modern, with nurses using all modern technology, but I came to this in a nursing home in rural England, and there was no need for any modern technology. It was all physical care. We ended up doing BBC – 'British Bottom Care'.

Another nurse, Sabita, whom I met in Scotland, said:[4] 'I did not know much about elderly care. I thought that we would get a job in an acute sector hospital as this is what nurses do in Nepal.'

The nature of nursing home work or residential care had been completely misunderstood by almost all the nurses I met and interviewed, and they had very different and unrealistic expectations. As Maya said:[5]

I did not know and understand the meaning of 'residential home'. When I received a letter that said I was to work in a nursing and residential home, I asked both the agent who arranged the work and my friend who was already working in a residential home for a further explanation. It was then explained by my Nepali friend that residential homes are where people live, get looked after and fed, etc. When I started working there I found it more like a hotel. I was supposed to be doing my adaptation training, but I was learning to set out the dinner trolley, offer and collect menus, serve food and feed elderly people, amongst many other things. It felt as if I was doing hotel management training, not learning any clinical nursing at all.

Maya worked in Nepal's oldest state-funded and, for Nepal, the most high-tech maternity hospital in Kathmandu, providing maternity services. She had further specialist training, and was used to managing maternity emergencies: dealing with all post-partum emergencies, setting up and starting intravenous fluid infusions and even giving emergency drugs. In her new job in a nursing home in England, however, she had to learn to take food orders and set up dinner tables. She thought that it was not necessary to be a trained nurse and experienced midwife to do the job she was now learning to do. She is just one of many, as Table 4.1 reveals. The nurses I interviewed had worked in the most technologically sophisticated areas like CCU, and others were in programme management level, before migrating to the UK. This is what they had expected to do in the UK. As Parvina said:[6] 'I thought nursing in the UK would be like the nursing we have observed and practised in Nepal, but only advanced [higher standard and technologically sophisticated]. I did not know anything about care of the elderly.'

This misunderstanding comes from Nepali nurses' lack of exposure to this type of work before they arrived in the UK. In Nepal, there are no nursing homes for long-term care and care of the elderly. Elderly people and people who need long-term care are looked after at home by their extended family members and relatives. Given the structure of most Nepali households it is mainly women, children and grandchildren who provide all support for the elderly. Modern technology and advances in healthcare systems, which help and support elderly and disabled people to live longer in western countries, are simply non-existent in Nepal. People may die of common illnesses and treatable conditions such as infections, so national health priorities and healthcare training focuses are very different.

Although private nursing homes have been operating since the late 1980s in Nepal, these are mainly in bigger urban centres like Kathmandu, Chitwan, Pokhara, Biratnagar, and Bhairahawa, but are not for care of the elderly. The services these nursing homes offer are very similar to the clinical services in private hospitals in the UK. Nepali nursing homes cater for wealthy clients with acute healthcare needs, including most types of medical, surgical and obstetric and gynaecological conditions. Due to the different population demography and different national health priorities, nursing plays a very small role in the care of the elderly and in rehabilitation settings, compared to the British healthcare scene. In Nepal mainstream nursing is geared mainly towards tertiary care services, as provided in major hospitals. Until 2006–2007, Nepali nurse education did not even focus in any way, either theoretically or practically, on the care of the elderly. This is a completely new area of nursing for Nepal-educated nurses, as was discussed in Chapter 1.

It can be seen that many Nepali nurses arrive in the UK with higher professional degrees and many years of experience. Not only do they possess advanced
qualifications and a great deal of experience, but they also hold high expectations. Their qualifications and experiences are not directly relevant to the nursing
jobs available for them in nursing homes; nevertheless, that is the setting in which
they find themselves. As Sumi explained above, they find the nature of long-term
care for the elderly, and disabled people in general, very basic and slow in pace.
It proves in essence to be deskilling. As Suruchi noted, nursing home work can
be described as 'BBC', and is clearly one of the least desired branches of nursing
in Britain (Adhikari & Melia 2013; Smith & Mackintosh 2007). When nurses
had to speak about the nature of their work in the UK, they appeared shy and
embarrassed. Many did not seem very keen to explain to me the nature of the
everyday work and share this with me. Some used alternative ways to tell people
what they do in a nursing home. For example, a Nepali carer (a nurse's husband)
I interviewed in East Sussex told me that his role was 'to provide pastoral care' to
nursing home residents but he would do many other things to help people,
'including feeding them and changing their clothes'.

While still in Nepal, nurses seem to imagine nursing in the West as technologically advanced, as it is advertised in nursing journals as a glamorous job;
quite the opposite to nursing home work. Some feel that a care home post is
just that of an assistant to people, requiring help with the activities of daily
living: feeding, washing and even just brushing people's hair. A senior nurse I
interviewed in the summer of 2007 in Nepal, who sounded like a potential
candidate for migration, said she wanted to verify some information with me:[7]

> I heard that nursing care jobs are easy in Britain, in America and in
> Australia. Patients there need help with having a shower, getting dressed
> and putting make-up on. Some women [elderly ladies] I heard want to
> have lipstick on, and help with food and sometimes with shopping, etc. I
> heard that they [elderly people] are lonely and don't live with their
> families, they need some companionship.

Hema, who I met in East Sussex, said she had experienced considerable sur-
prise when she went to work in a nursing home for the first time:[8] 'Before
coming here, my expectations were that I would get very good work in a big
hospital, very busy, hard work – a luxurious place to work, with a good
salary, all computerised, etc.'

But once she started working, she realised the truth of her new situation:

> I was in a small nursing home. The care there was good but there was not
> enough opportunity to learn much about clinical nursing [not exposed to
> many clinical activities and nursing procedures] ... I did not get clinical
> nursing experience, I did not get the chance to get exposure to many
> areas [of acute care nursing], and I did not even get the chance to learn
> about wound dressing.

Care of the elderly, or geriatric nursing, is seen by many as 'basic care'. Melia has illustrated how even nursing students in Britain considered this type of nursing, to be 'not really nursing' but basic care (Melia 1987: 132–135). For many of these Nepali nurses, who do not share the same cultural background as the people they look after, it is not surprising that they consider this branch of long-term care nursing as being basic, slow and menial and, understandably for them too, not really nursing.

Workload

Not only was the type of nursing a shock, but many nurses also perceived the workload in nursing homes to be very heavy. Many admitted that they were not used to this amount of work in Nepal. Kiran said:[9]

> but when I arrived here, it was all about only pad round [changing diapers regularly], basic wash, feeding people and putting them in bed. I found it completely different from what I had thought. What happened at first was the *Didi* [older sister] I had lived with said one day, OK, come with me, I will take you to my nursing home. In a nursing home in Nepal, they have young adults and old people and children and all in general. Nepali nursing homes are big and modern. But, here they are only for old people. I went to that nursing home with her, she took me to an elderly woman. She was so skinny. When I saw her, I was terrified as she only had skin and bone in her body. A few minutes later she took me to another woman who was over 100 kilos. I was thinking, how can you look after that person? And she says we have to lift them up, she says, and, we have to put them in bed, feed them wash them, etc. When I heard about looking after old people, I thought it would be old people like our old folks in Nepal, who can walk about and go to bed and get up all by themselves, but here it is very different. It is almost 90 per cent different from what I had imagined. I thought that I would be working in a ward, and like that. There is a vast difference from what I had thought.

A nurse's husband in Aberdeen told me:[10]

> My wife regularly cries after doing a long day in a nursing home, she says it is too hard and too tiring, how long can she last like this. She tells me that nurses and carers have to deal with very heavily dependent residents.

Sumi, in Scotland, said:

> Usually we are always short of staff. Eh … staff–patient ratio. It would look OK until somebody phones off sick. In the morning, there would be one or two registered nurses and the manager plus four carers; and in the evening one registered nurse and three carers for 25 to 30 residents. But

regularly staff phone to report they are off sick. If all staff came on duty, the staff–patient ratio would be OK. But ... it's like that everywhere, when they feel tired and get lazy and don't want to go to work they phone in sick, this is a common problem in a nursing home. The rest of the staff will have an extra workload as there is nobody available to replace these sick. For example, it is like this as it depends on their mood ... in a little while if I don't want to go to work, I too will phone them and tell them that I am not well ... [She giggles] But I have never done this myself.

As the example above reveals, if shortages of staff occur in the nursing home setting, perhaps due to sickness, personnel are not replaced. Work is accordingly divided amongst the available staff there and then. Nursing home work is already viewed as heavy, but nurses regularly have to share this extra workload. These practical issues are difficult to understand when nurses are still in Nepal. The nurses' experiences described above, particularly regarding the practical and everyday nature of nursing home work and the workload, did not seem to be fed back to nurses in Nepal at the time. When I asked Sara what she would share with her nurse friends in Nepal about her work environment and workload, if they wanted to come to Britain, she replied:[11]

I will tell all the truth about the nature of nursing care [referring to the nature of nursing and workload] in Britain to my friends, if they still want to come and do the job that is fine ... at least they are informed about it.

Sara too had gone through a period of extreme frustration and disappointment, but at the time of interview was settled in a proper staff nurse post. Whether she will tell the whole story in Nepal is another issue, and one to which I will return later in this chapter.

In summary, before migrating to the UK, Nepali nurses had neither training nor socio-cultural exposure to care of the elderly and long-term care settings, so their initial experiences have not been positive or fulfilling. As time passes, however, nursing home work in Britain becomes more normal and more acceptable to them. Like Sumi, nurses come to realise that there is no easy way for them to find their dream job, and like it or not, many are compelled to accept nursing home jobs. After coming to terms with this, most nurses seem to focus on working as many hours as possible, and earning as much money as they physically can. Their goalposts have had to be moved and, at least for a while, their main aim now becomes to save money. For those who have been separated from their families, family reunion is their next major goal. This will depend on the nurses' savings, so the availability of working hours and monthly earnings become very important. Despite the undesirable nature of nursing home work and the heavy workload, many nurses are prepared to work for as many hours as they can.

Working hours and money

The majority of the nurses I interviewed, between 2007 and 2009, were working night shifts and unsocial hours. Some were working in more than one place. I was told this was a necessity, in order to become financially viable in Britain; to recover from debt; and try to repay the money they had borrowed and invested when making their move to the UK. Those who planned to bring their family here needed to have 'a good bank balance' and a regular monthly income, and so their energies seemed to be concentrated towards these goals. When I enquired about their achievements and successes, almost everybody said that their main achievement had been the number of working hours and the total amount of money they were able to earn each month. Many expressed the view that 'good' hours are working 60, 70 and sometimes even 80 hours a week. In every interview, the nurses' immediate responses about their hours were either 'Yes: *Majjako Hours Paienchha* [one gets plenty of hours]', or 'No: *Hoursnai Paindaina* [one does not get enough hours]'. The following conversation illustrates this:[12]

EVA: I am happy here, *Majjako Hours Paienchha* [good or plenty of hours are available] and I have to be happy with this.

RADHA: Then you were in Oxford. It was alright there you said, and there too you were getting 'good hours'?

EVA: Yes, then in Oxford. It was OK. But we did not get paid so well there, as we were sent by the agency: they used to take money off from our hourly rate to pay the agency. We only received £5.35 an hour. Because this nursing home had to pay the agency fee that money came from our salary, we were told. They [agents] used to get commission from our salary too. Those who work more hours earn more and those who work fewer hours earn less ... right from the start I have been very lucky, I have not had any problem with getting *Majjako Hours* – good number of hours.

Eva had left her husband and two children in Nepal. When I met her in London in summer 2007, she was trying hard to save up as much money as she could, so that she would be able to invite her family to join her. For many Nepali nurses, as with many low-paid workers, working long hours becomes more of a necessity than a choice, in order to increase their chances of reuniting with their families.

Namrata informed me that she moved to the UK in July 2005. At the time of the interview (in spring 2008) she seemed quite settled. She said that initially she worked very hard and for many hours a week, on regular nights and double shifts, so that she could earn enough to repay the loan she took out to move to the UK and also help her elderly mother in Nepal. When I met her in East Sussex, she was working at night, and doing some long days too. She had her two children with her there, and she said she was happy with her achievements so far.

Most nurses work extra hours purely to support their families and their husbands' or their children's education. One nurse who worked in a nursing home, in a small village near Bath, told me:[13]

> My son is at university here in England. I am paying for his overseas student's rate that is around £10,000 a year. I have to work longer hours and extra days some weeks just to survive and pay his fees.

Another nurse, who came to the UK in 2008 as a dependent wife, started to look for a job soon after she arrived. Her husband was an international full fee-paying student, at a cost to them of over £9,000 a year. In order to repay the money they borrowed to make the initial investment for migration, she had to work longer hours every day. She said:[14]

> The nursing home does not pay any extra money for working unsocial hours or in the weekend. The rates are not very good so I have to work more hours. Some weeks I work 50 and 60 hours, usually 12 hours a day from 8 a.m. to 8 p.m. I have never worked like this before in Nepal, and I get very tired and I feel like crying sometimes. But I don't have much choice.

Many nurses do not receive unsocial hours allowances in private nursing homes. They have to work many hours to survive and support their families here. Some employers even produce fake documents for nurses to show to the Home Office in order to secure a work permit. Some will even fake nurses' salaries and other benefits. Maya received a job offer and a fake contract to work in a nursing home in London. She informed me:[15]

> The manager at my new job in London has forwarded my work permit document which says my post would be the Deputy Manager for this care home with a salary of over £22,000, but I will get paid about £18,000 a year. It is easier to get a work permit as a deputy manager than as an ordinary staff nurse.

This arrangement was perhaps a win-win situation for both parties involved: vulnerable employees find jobs and get extra hours of work and employers benefit from a cheap workforce, but it is also a clear example of manipulation of UK immigration and employment regulations.

A common phenomenon is that all nurses need to work as many hours as possible, irrespective of their initial visa status. Many who came to the UK to do NVQ courses have to pay their fees for these courses and their visa extensions. Nurses' long working hours are clearly illustrated by Usha, whom I interviewed in East Sussex in the summer of 2008. I had arranged an interview with Usha in early April, and had difficulty in finding a mutually suitable time for this. I was there for four days, and all that time she was working. She told me that she tried to work many hours a week in a series of nursing homes in the area, and she was very tired. She had left her husband and two children in Nepal and was desperately trying to save up, and bring her family over to the UK as soon as she could. The day before I was to leave East Sussex, I managed to get some time with her, but only after 8 p.m., and we met in her flat. She was living in a shared house with four other Nepalis, three of whom were also nurses. I arrived a little early and spoke with another nurse. Usha arrived during a conversation about working and living in England, and told me that she had to go to London the next morning. She spoke of how tired and busy she was, but that she was happy to talk to me.

Usha had worked a night shift the night before, returning to her flat in the morning for a couple of hours sleep only, as she was booked to work an evening shift in a different nursing home. I met her after that shift and the next day would have been her only free day that week, but she had to go to London to sort out her student visa status, as her current visa was about to expire. She had to go to a college in East London to enrol on an Information Technology (IT) course. She revealed to me later that she managed that relatively easily, as she knew an agent there who helped her obtain all the necessary documents. She had to pay a fee for this service as well as the course fee, and she was then ready to apply for a student visa extension. When she returned to her flat in the evening, she said that she was absolutely exhausted, and had a long day shift booked for the next day. She worked as many hours as she could in that home, as there was no guarantee of work for the day after next and for the next week. She mentioned that she had not seen her six- and nine-year-old sons for two years. She would speak to them on the phone regularly, and she would instruct her husband how to look after the children. She said that she missed them very much, but she was doing all this for her family and for the children's future, hoping that soon they would be reunited. Many nurses worked like Usha to save enough money in their bank accounts to satisfy visa officers into granting their families dependants' visas.

Another nurse in East Sussex revealed:[16]

> We came here to work, so I have to work. Some weeks I work 60, 70 and I have worked up to 80 hours in a week. I have to do this to support my family and to survive here. I am hoping to invite my sons here soon.

Having explored the initial culture shock the nurses experienced at their workplace, I next consider the working relationships nurses have had with their colleagues, patients/residents, patients' relatives and their line managers.

Working relationships with people at work

New staff members in any working environment need to be socially integrated and fully accepted by their colleagues, in order to establish good working relationships. For many internationally educated nurses, however, racial discrimination and harassment at work is a barrier to this. In many instances, the existing workforce does not welcome new migrant nurses as a part of the team, leading inevitably to feelings of exclusion. Sumi has described, in detail, her poor working relationship with her colleagues and line manager. This kind of racism and discrimination at work has been one of the most widely reported and discussed experiences of migrant nurses globally, as well as being the subject of extensive research. Kingma (2006) presents some examples of British nurses experiencing racism/harassment and discrimination in Australia, and Jamaican nurses encountering similar experiences in the USA. There has been considerable research and discussion on internationally educated and black and minority ethnic nurses being victims of discrimination in the UK healthcare system (Dalphinis 2007; Larsen 2007; Smith et al. 2006; Winklemann-Gleed 2006; RCN 2007).

Racism and discrimination are experienced in different forms and expressed in various ways. Sumi's account of being the target of bullying in her workplace was just another example of how poorly migrant nurses can be treated. Some nurses felt that patients, and their relatives, preferred to be looked after by 'white' nurses, recognising this as a further form of racial discrimination. Nurses shared their experiences with me, and the following unpacks the different presentations of racism they encountered at work, starting with their relationships with the patients they were caring for, then their patients' relatives, before finally moving to a discussion of their relationships with colleagues and line managers.

Relationship with patients and their relatives

Maya, who had informed me of not even understanding the meaning of 'residential home' before coming to Britain, explained that it can be very humiliating when residents and their relatives do not accept migrant staff, and fail to regard them as qualified and skilled professionals. She had regularly experienced a measure of rejection from service-users and had witnessed her work colleagues suffering in similar circumstances. She gave this example:[17]

> A retired elderly man who worked in the Air Force during the war, he used to shout out loud and said 'where am I, where am I?' I told him that he was in England, in a nursing home near his family home. He said 'It does not feel like that, there are so many black people here' … this nursing home is staffed heavily by migrant care workers, we have Indian, Sri Lankan, Polish and other European [including herself, a Nepali] staff in this nursing home.

She made the further point that establishing a trusting and good working relationship with work colleagues and patients' relatives was also very challenging. Other nurses also expressed how hard it was to earn trust and recognition from patients' relatives, and one told of her frustration with this problem:[18]

> This probably does not happen to you [indicating me as a nurse]. It is very hard to establish a good working relationship with relatives and families. I'll give you an example. I was working in a nursing home one afternoon. I have a full nursing registration [NMC PIN], I was the only qualified nurse on the ward, and I was in-charge for the shift. In the afternoon, relatives and families came to see patients, some of them walking past me went straight to talk to a carer, a white staff member to find out about a patient and how she had been over the last few days, etc. They would not come to me but they bypassed me and went straight to a carer. I felt it was not the qualification or experience they [relatives] were interested in but the skin colour of the staff.

Although these examples indicate that migrant nurses can be subtly and overtly rejected by nursing home residents and their relatives, not many nurses openly and voluntarily mentioned that they found difficulty establishing and maintaining relationships with patients, possibly because their working relationships with patients and relatives may seem like a secondary issue compared to the many other major challenges migrant nurses have to face at work. Perhaps because of the patients' dependency, elderly and vulnerable people are not usually in a position to question nurses' actions, or perhaps it does not happen so often. But when a patient does comment, they can sound fairly severe, as Maya felt above. A stressful working relationship with colleagues and managers, however, was more frequently mentioned and by many nurses.

Relationship with colleagues and managers

Sumi said her manager always tried to be politically correct, and started conversations by saying 'a very good friend of mine is Indian', before moving into 'this is how we do things here' in a subtly undermining and twisted way, before becoming personally critical. Sumi felt people at work had various types of racist behaviours, not all of them totally transparent and easy to explain. Her manager harassed her in a very subtle and 'politically correct' manner, by trying to present herself as a non-racist and a rather friendly person, who had an Indian friend. Although the manager sought to cloak her discriminatory behaviour, her treatment of Sumi was tantamount to racial harassment. Some other nurses felt 'watched' or 'policed' by their local colleagues and these experiences were commonly felt and are described by many (Henry 2008; Allan & Larsen 2003; Winkelmann-Gleed 2006). This type of working relationship served to exclude migrant nurses from work-related socialisation. Many nurses told me informally that they had started isolating themselves from engagements with work colleagues, given their feelings of exclusion.

Nurses regularly felt discriminated against. Errors made by local staff members were dealt differently to those made by migrant nurses. Hema, working in East Sussex, had an image of British people as very friendly, which she gathered from some British people she had met in Nepal before coming to the UK. But when she started working in London, she realised that not all were as she had imagined them. She further reported witnessing local nurses hiding and covering up colleagues' weaknesses and mistakes, but that migrant nurses were treated differently:[19]

HEMA: I had met some British people in Nepal and I thought that they all would be very polite, friendly, all very nice, very kind, and caring. But I found only 2–3 per cent of people like that. The rest are *jealous, back-biting, dirty talking, swearing, racist* [with emphasis] like that. There are a few nice people, too, but racism is a major problem. I have this frustration. There are a few very nice people, too, but the majority of them are racist, some can be nice to your face but stab you in the back. If a local [white] makes any complaint against a foreign staff member, the manager would listen, the managers would listen to local white, but if a foreigner makes any similar complaint they all get together and isolate the person who complained, and gang-up against the foreign staff. So there is very little point to make any complaint.

RADHA: ... they would listen to complaints made by locals, but not by the foreigners? Can you explain it a bit more, please?

HEMA: ... for example, the place where I work now, there are European staff and non-European staff. If a local makes a complaint against a migrant the manager would listen and take action against the migrant [nurse]. But, if a migrant does the same, the manager would gang-up with the staff [local] and isolate the person who makes the complaint. Because of this, many migrants and mainly Asian nurses do not go to the manager with any issue. This is totally frustrating. I have seen this happening to my friends, so it feels like it can happen to me as well. Sometimes it is so frustrating; they cover up the mistakes made by the English staff.

Hema and a few of her colleagues discovered that there were some drug errors and drug misuse in her nursing home and thought they knew the perpetrator. The manager took no action and it was covered up very quickly. At this point Hema asked me to turn my recorder off, before a further exploration of this, as she did not feel comfortable about recording it all.

Smith et al.'s study (2006) also shows that some healthcare managers react differently to mistakes made by migrant nurses, compared with home-trained nurses.

Occupational socialising: language and culture as barriers

On the whole, having a common language and a shared culture makes socialising at work easier. Migrant nurses are disadvantaged in coming from different socio-cultural backgrounds, and having a lack of proficiency in English (Winklemann-Gleed 2006; Smith et al. 2006). Although most of the Nepali nurses I met spoke very good English, they have found many of their British counterparts very unwelcoming and exclusive. Some felt that their main weakness was English language. Kiran, in East Sussex, said:[20]

> Our communication skill is poor. However hard we try, people here do not understand our accent. We have communication problem, this is the main problem. For example, from when I was young, I spoke with British and had English medium education [went to an English-medium private school in Nepal]. I worked in Nepal with British people too. It is quite different to communicate here with a mass, from communicating there with an individual. This is our main weakness, communicating here ... some staff members try hard to understand us, but the residents and the visitors they don't understand us; I feel this is our main weakness.

This is perhaps a barrier to socialising at work, but it is a barrier created, as well as fuelled, by the current institutional regulations in the UK, with discriminatory practice imposed by the UK nursing regulatory body, the NMC. Its policy states it is important that all nurses should be able to communicate clearly and effectively with their clients and colleagues at work. The NMC, however, has a double set of rules for overseas nurses, depending on the nurses' nationality: from the EU vs. from outside the EU. The already cited demand for nurses from outwith EU countries to achieve IELTS score 7, in each aspect of English, is in itself discriminatory, for it is not deemed necessary for nurses coming from Spain, France, Poland or elsewhere in Europe. If nurses are to offer a good standard of nursing care to people, either all nurses from non-English speaking backgrounds need IELTS scores of 7 or they do not. There should be one professional standard, which does not depend on a nurse's nationality. This type of institutional discrimination, and regulation based on nationality, only serves to increase Nepali nurses' feelings of vulnerability, and to make them feel their status is weaker than that of EU nurses, and that their practical nursing skills and caring attitudes are not taken into any account at work. Overseas nurses' competency is assessed by the NMC against their nationality and English ability, not their clinical skills and caring and compassionate qualities.

Cultural differences can also play an important role in nurses' socialisation. Amongst the Nepali nurses I met and interviewed, some follow Hinduism and some Christianity, and some do not practise religion at all. One Hindu nurse commented that she still does not eat beef, as the cow is a holy animal for Hindus in Nepal. She did not want to share a flat or kitchen with her work colleagues, as they would eat beef, and she did not feel comfortable even going out with them for the evening.[21] Religion and culture appeared to be important issues impacting on some nurses' social lives.

Dealing with racial issues at work

After recognising that racism, discrimination, and harassment at work exist widely, in 2005, the RCN UK developed 'RCN good practice guidance for employers in recruiting and retaining' overseas nurses within the Working Well Initiative (RCN 2005). This good practice guide suggests that employers offer some degree of orientation and training for local nurses about the situation of overseas nurses, in order to enable better social integration, and to build a good working environment and an effective team. This is certainly a noble idea, but it appears not to have been translated into everyday practice. The British NHS is an equal opportunity employer in theory only, given that many migrant staff have continued to experience racism from their colleagues, managers, patients and relatives.

The RCN and UNISON are the main trade union bodies for nurses in the UK. They are trying to raise awareness of migrant nurses' issues to promote social and professional integration. Since 2002 in particular, when the British media started to expose the exploitation of overseas nurses in Britain (BBC News 2005; Red Pepper 2004; BBC News 2002) both organisations have been actively involved in advocacy and lobbying work to improve the working environment for overseas as well as black and minority ethnic (BME) nurses.[22] The RCN and UNISON have regional branches in various parts of the country, with a network group for overseas nurses, designed to facilitate better support for them.[23] Not all migrant nurses are members, however. I interviewed a nurse in East Sussex who was opposed to joining either of these bodies, first because the membership fee was too expensive (about £15 per month for full membership, in 2007) and second because she did not have much faith in them. She echoed Sumi's experience in her description of discriminatory practices in the British healthcare system as being sometimes so subtle that even such a powerful body as the RCN can do little to tackle them. In short, nurses' trade union organisations have failed to be fully effective in combating the problems.

Migrant nurses and career progression opportunities

As discussed, during the initial fieldwork I had met many nurses struggling to find permanent nursing jobs and work permits. Some had just found a permanent position, and some were desperately trying to find training placements. They were looking for some job security first, and were not that well paid either. None of the nurses' past qualifications and experience had been recognised or were being valued in the UK, so all had started from the bottom of the UK professional ladder. Career progression was not a major issue for the majority, as they were preoccupied with other pressing issues. However, as Table 4.1 suggests, after a period of career setback in their early years in the UK, some nurses have made reasonable progress in their professional careers: some have gone on to higher level studies, others are working in the NHS, having secured Permanent Residency. Some have remained in the nursing home sector and a small number have returned to Nepal.

There is plenty of available research literature suggesting that migrant nurses do not get the jobs for which they are fully qualified and have the experience to do. In terms of promotion opportunities, even in the NHS, where working terms and conditions are considerably better than in private sector nursing homes, many overseas nurses experience career stagnation (Kline 2014; RCN 2007; Smith et al. 2006; Winklemann-Gleed 2006; Allan & Larsen 2003). Overseas nurses have to be exceptionally good to be shortlisted for, or be offered any sought-after, or longed-for, promoted post. Career promotion opportunities in private nursing homes are far fewer for nurses from ethnic minority backgrounds.

Conclusion

This chapter has demonstrated that many Nepali nurses come to the UK with very unrealistic work expectations. They bring with them work experience in very different types of nursing posts from the ones in which they find themselves employed in the UK. It has also illustrated that Nepali nurses' expertise and qualifications are not valued, and consequently their experience and skills are misplaced in the British healthcare system. For the majority of nurses from Nepal, migration to the UK means a downward professional move, as is the case for other migrant nurses (Larsen 2007). After leaving a successful professional career behind, they come to the UK and take up the very least desired type of nursing and in suboptimal working environments. Many have experienced work-related culture shock. Nurses' salaries and benefits are not very attractive, and some are not even paid unsocial working hours enhancements. Despite difficult working relationships with colleagues, and regularly feeling rejected by patients and patients' relatives, many nurses are forced by their circumstances to work extra shifts whenever any opportunity is available. Compared to the working terms and conditions in private nursing homes, the NHS does offer a better deal for migrant nurses. However, nurses have to wait before a move to the NHS sector, as they have to achieve 'Permanent Residency' status first, which takes five years of working full-time with a work permit. They also have to wait, patiently again, for their family to be reunited, and for any further education and professional development opportunities. How they navigate, and have navigated all these further challenges, is discussed in the next chapter.

Notes

1 Nursing homes and residential care homes in the UK provide personal and nursing care to elderly and disabled people. Generally, people come to these institutions for long-term care, and it is not often that they get better and go home. For many overseas nurses this is a totally new social phenomenon (RCN 2005).

2 Interviewed in East Sussex, England, February 2008.

3 Interview in rural Oxfordshire, England, March 2007. The first time I heard the expression 'BBC' or 'British Bottom Care' was from a Nepali nurse, but this expression was widely used by migrant nurses from other countries, mainly those who work in private nursing homes (Allan and Larsen 2003; Smith et al. 2006).

4 Interviewed in Dundee, Scotland, June 2007.

5 Interviewed in rural Northumberland, England, May 2007.

6 Interviewed in Dundee, Scotland, June 2007.

7 Interviewed (a nurse lecturer) in Kathmandu, Nepal, July 2008.

8 Interviewed in East Sussex, England, April 2008.

9 Interviewed in East Sussex, England, February 2008.

10 Conversation (with a nurse's husband) in Edinburgh, Scotland, June 2009.

11 Interviewed in Buckinghamshire, England, February 2007.

12 Interviewed in London, England, April 2007. I had a telephone conversation with one of Eva's friends in spring 2009 and was informed that Eva had been joined by her husband and their two children, and they were living in London.

13 Telephone conversation with Tala, May 2009; she then lived in a small village near Bath, England.

14 Conversation in Edinburgh, Scotland, March 2009.

15 Interviewed in rural Northumberland, England, May 2007.

16 Interviewed in East Sussex, England, April 2008.

17 Interviewed in rural Northumberland, England, May 2007.

18 Interviewed in Dundee, Scotland, May 2007.

19 Interviewed in East Sussex, England, April 2008.

20 Interviewed in East Sussex, England, February 2008.

21 Since I considered religious belief to be a private matter, I did not actively explore the nurses' religious beliefs and practices, although if they had an issue or wanted to express something they could do so.

22 Information on their activities can be found in their websites: www.rcn.org.uk and www.unison.org.uk, both accessed on 7/4/2019.

23 There was an overseas nurses' network group in Edinburgh, set up in 2005. It remained active for a couple of years but recently has been very quiet. As an overseas nurse and a researcher, I am still a member, though the group has been inactive for a while.

5 Negotiating with new realities
Family and social lives in the UK

One of the main reasons why Nepali nurses who took part in this study wanted to move the UK was to work in a fully resourced and high-tech healthcare system, enjoy a higher living standard and start a better future for their children and other family members. The previous chapter has illustrated how disappointed they were with their working conditions, as their high hopes were dashed and their dreams were unfulfilled. This chapter examines their experience of family and social life in the UK: their living situations, how they and their families re-adjusted and adapted to their new environment. It will question whether they found the higher living standard they sought, and a final focus will be on what their social support networks were in the UK. The chapter concludes with a discussion of the overall migration experience of nurses, their new hopes and dreams, and the adjustment strategies they have developed for a better future.

Living situations and social lives

Nepali nurses and their families in the UK live and work in diverse locations: from major urban centres like London to rural settings. Cities offer larger social networks with many living near their friends, and some even house or flat-sharing. Others seem to have created and joined small Nepali communities and close social support networks.

The exact number is not available but there has been a significant increase in the Nepali migrant population in the UK since 2001; from around 5,000 in 2001 to almost 50,000 in 2008 (Sims 2008), and this number has continued to grow in the last decade. Several new Nepali diaspora networks have emerged: ethnicity based, profession based, and locality or geography based, which is explored in more detail later in this chapter. Most Nepalis live in and around London and Southeast England, organising various cultural events and functions, and taking part in major Nepali festivals and socio-cultural rituals.

A snapshot of nurses and their families, in April 2008, is revelatory of the growth of the diaspora. Several hundred nurses (and many with their families) were living in London; 35 nurses and their families were in Hastings; with several nurses and their families in Reading, Watford, Harrow-on-the-Hill, and in Oxfordshire. In Aberdeen there were ten to 12 nurses and five in and around Dundee. The majority were living in small clusters. It is important to note that these are only a small sample of possible locations in the UK where I have been reliably informed Nepalis are living. I was unable to visit many of the rural locations, nor the cities of Southampton, Eastbourne, Liverpool and Manchester; and several towns in East Anglia, North Wales and Belfast in Northern Ireland.

I visited Hastings and St Leonards several times, between 2007 and 2015, meeting nurses and their families, living in clusters of two to three families in a house, with two to three such households in one street. I was informed that similar clusters existed in Charlton and Woolwich, Southeast London, and in West London in Wembley, Southall, Watford and Harrow on-the-Hill. Some nurses in Hastings and St Leonards were living in the town but working in rural nursing homes, ten to 12 miles outside Hastings, but within commuting distance. Hema, for example, was working several miles from town in a rural nursing home, albeit one with a regular train service, but chose to live in Hastings itself for the social network and support, and for her children to socialise with other Nepali families.

Many other nurses were rurally based too, across the UK, appearing socially quite 'cut off' from other Nepalis, and in fact expressing feelings of isolation. When I visited some of the nursing homes deep in the countryside, there was very limited public transport: very infrequent services especially in the evenings and at weekends. These nurses did not have their own transport and seemed completely isolated and almost trapped in their villages. They were often the only Nepali nurse or family in the village, so little happened outside work and school. Children lacked friends with whom to play and husbands were not able to find proper jobs, so felt isolated and lonely.

I visited Sara, who was living in nursing home accommodation (in an attic room in the same nursing home building, which was a little dark but self-contained and comfortable) in rural Buckinghamshire, about 15 miles outside Oxford, near Bicester. We arranged to meet at 4 p.m. after her day shift. I planned to be there for around 4.30 p.m., but found there was no transport available and had to take a taxi from Bicester, only to discover that there would be no public transport of any kind after 5 p.m. When I was ready to return to Oxford I had difficulty in finding even a taxi. Sara said that because of this lack of transport she could not go out very often, neither to Oxford itself or any nearby town. She went food shopping once a week but she had no flexibility about this, as to miss the last bus would have caused her considerable difficulty.

Another nurse, Indra, with whom I spoke on the telephone in March 2009, and have met several times since then, said she had been living and working in a rural nursing home in Lancashire since coming to England in 2004, her husband and children having joined her in 2006. She told me her family were the only Nepali people in this village in the heart of English countryside, almost an hour's bus journey from Preston. They hardly saw any other Nepalis for months, and she had no Nepali friend there, so she spent her time either working in a nursing home or with her family. With so little happening in the village for her children, they spent many hours on the computer every day.[1]

Wherever they are, in general, migrants usually live in poor and cramped housing conditions. Some accommodation is provided as part of a work contract, but this is usually more expensive than the ordinary going rate (Castle 2000; Shelley 2007). If a nurse is new in the country and with no other social support, she has little choice but to accept, and try to be thankful for, whatever is available. Nepali nurses' situations are no exception. I have witnessed many nurses' living conditions and accommodation and they matched the description of Castle (2000) and Shelley (2007): rundown, rough, cramped and overpriced. Some nurses who had recently arrived in Britain told me that their employers had arranged their accommodation, but at a premium rates. Rents seemed unreasonably expensive. I met nurses in East Sussex, Oxfordshire and Scotland, who were sharing a house with other migrant nurses and, in many instances, it emerged that their nursing home employer owned the property. In urban hubs or in isolated rural areas, wherever they were, most of the nurses' accommodation I visited did seem quite rundown, and some nurses were living in worryingly rough parts of towns.

Witness an incident when I was in St Leonard's on Sea near Hastings, and making the five-minute walk, from one house to another nurse's house. It was late morning when I encountered a group of rough-looking young people near the local train station, some of whom seemed already to be drunk. With no other pedestrians around, I felt unsafe and I ran quickly. However I realised that, if I had to live there, I would not be able to walk around freely in the evenings or at night. Nurses living there reported that they usually asked their husbands and friends to escort them to and from work, with it being an essential precaution in the evening and at night.

Whether in a tranquil rural village or an urban hub such as Hastings, in a 'mini Nepali village', wherever nurses lived, many have found their social lives restricted and very different from their dreams and hopes of life in the UK. Their social lives were restricted for a number of reasons. First, as we have seen in the previous chapter, many nurses worked many extra hours a week (over the recommended full-time hours of 37.5 a week for the NHS) and had no free time. Second, many did not have families in the UK, having initially travelled solo, and they sorely missed their families and loved ones. Finally, many found the business of making new friends in a new place very challenging, because of cultural and language differences.

Gradually, however, migrant nurses started to seek out better social networks, as well as better jobs. When these opportunities arose, nurses moved to be near their friends and families. Sumi, whom I introduced in the previous chapter, moved to a Scottish town to be near her relatives. In March 2008, two other nurses moved up to rural Scotland, accompanied by their families. One nurse had found a job and, after settling there, invited her friend to follow in her footsteps. Within a few months her friend managed to secure a post in the same nursing home and moved to be near her: a form of chain migration.

Social life: also a delusion

We first met Kiran[2] in Chapter 2. She had explained how unrealistic her expectations of working as a nurse in the UK had turned out to be. She had, she said, also entertained a completely wrong idea about Nepali nurses and their social lives in Britain. The images she had had were nothing like the reality and she admitted to having been very deluded. She giggled as she told me this, appearing slightly embarrassed to share her personal feelings openly. She used to receive holiday photos from a close friend, who had migrated to London with her husband in the mid-1990s. Her friend's husband was a British Gurkha. She spoke of the photos and what they had meant to her then:

> Here she used to send us photos, always looking very pleasant and happy. She only sent happy-looking photos ... [giggle]. She used to stay in Lewisham in London. Quite a lot of Nepalis lived there. She sent us photos of *Teej, Dasai* and *Tihar* [major Nepali Hindu festivals]. And she lived near her family and relations, so photos with her *Didi-Bahini* and *Daju-Bhai*, like that. All looking happy, always on holiday, like they never knew about any difficulty. So I had prepared myself and aspired for that kind of life. Their photos of wearing expensive *saris* and so much gold jewellery like that, it all looked very nice.

Kiran told me that, on seeing the photos, she wished to be there too, but it felt almost like a dream to her then. 'I thought if we get to go to the UK, we all will have a fantastic life, happy in a society with higher living standards and working in a technologically advanced system.'

Although her friend was also working as a carer in a nursing home, one thing she had never mentioned, or shared with others, was her working situation and her social life. Kiran could not really understand what it would be like to work and live in the UK, and her friend's photos did not really give her a full picture of that work or social life. Once here in the UK, Kiran found that the social life quite different to that which she had imagined: 'We don't get time to see even our close friends much, so I have no social life or a very restricted one.'

Kiran lived in East Sussex, with many Nepali nurses and their families nearby. As such, she was in a better position than many others. She even shared a house with another Nepali couple. Nevertheless she still found her social life restricted, and for many of the nurses living rurally, their social lives felt extremely confined.

I met Maya and her family in rural village in Northern England.[3] They were the only Nepali family there and did not find their social lives stimulating in that setting. She said that she had almost no contact with other Nepalis when she first arrived there in 2004.

After arriving in London on her own, Maya was sent to this rural location, where she completed her adaptation training. When we met in May 2007, she had been living in that village for almost three years: the first two on her own, and the third year with her family. She shared her initial experience of living in the village, having left her family back in Nepal and with no Nepali friend nearby. She said:

> I used to work usually six to seven days a week initially, sometimes long days [12-hour shifts] ... and after the shift I had no social life. I would work in a nursing home, come home after the shift, then nothing, no family here and no friends nearby. I was desperately missing my family. I lived on my own for two full years, and I lost so much weight, I was getting much thinner. I used to write and post letters, and I used to go to the village post office. There is nothing in the village, one church, one pub, a local shop and a post office. The post office was closed down a few years ago; after this I felt that there was nothing in the village left for me. Food and other items are very expensive here. I went to Newcastle a few times to meet up with other Nepalis. There was nobody to talk to or do anything with or any activity at all in the village. I felt so lonely and with no social life I started going to the village church. My family joined me a year ago, it is better for me now.

Living in this village on her own Maya had clearly missed her family terribly. Despite feeling so lonely and isolated she had no option but to stay there. She could not make friends there, and feeling so dispirited and isolated, she did not bother to cook for herself, or eat regular meals, hence her considerable weight loss. She had even tried going to the local church a few times to see if she could meet and talk to someone, but with little success. She found making friends and socialising in a village quite challenging. She felt that anybody from outside the village was seen as a migrant, and was treated, by the community, as if he/she was from different planet.

Reshaping a new social life: a challenge

All migrants have to restart their lives in a strange society. Creating a support network in a new society is not always easy, and it has not been easy for Nepali nurses in the UK. As Maya's story above suggests, socio-cultural differences make it harder for newcomers to integrate with locals in an alien place. New food customs and religious practices may be some of the differences encountered on the way, as people journey to becoming gradually assimilated into a new, and increasingly multicultural, society in the UK.

Some of the differences might seem relatively small, but they affect nurses in their everyday lives and in social integration processes.

Other and more prominent barriers to socialising with work colleagues and local people pertain. Sumi, who I introduced in Chapter 4, had lived on her own and, it was difficult for her to mix with her neighbours and work colleagues in a small Scottish town. She sadly expressed:[4]

> Yes, social life. I thought that it would be different. In a foreign country, I had higher expectations of living standards and social life. Sometimes it seems like I am in Nepal, as the living standard is not different, now I am sure that I was day-dreaming on that day and thinking that I was in Nepal. It does not seem strange or a high standard where I live now. Just a few days ago, I was at work, a person with blonde hair walked in, I thought this person is in Nepal, has come to visit Nepal. For a second I thought that this person was a tourist in Nepal. I must have got completely lost [she giggles]. When I first arrived I went to Eastbourne, there I spent so much time with other Asians, and it did not feel like Britain at all, I did not get any chance to learn about social life in Britain. Then I moved here [Scotland]. Here too I don't socialise with the locals or work colleagues, I don't interact with them. I am not like that, sometimes they invite me for a night out, and I don't go ... If you don't go once or twice, they would not invite you again. I am not that kind of person ... I got invited out a few times but I did not go so they don't invite me again ... I go out with work colleagues only for work related stuff that is all. I have no personal relationships ...

RADHA: So, you don't mix with the local work colleagues much. What do you do on your day off, or in your holidays, how do you spend your time? You said that you sleep a lot – apart from that?

SUMI: I sleep a lot, sleep until about 10–11 in the morning, when I am not working. I invite my *Dai*, *Didi* and friends, whoever is there and is free to come online [in Nepal] when I am free here to chat online. I watch television. I go to the library and borrow a film and watch it. Sometimes I go and see my Nepali friends and other times I watch DVDs or just sleep.

As the interview progressed, Sumi further revealed that she did not want to socialise with her work colleagues; she would rather spend time chatting with her friends and families in Nepal and with friends who have migrated internationally. Socialising with locals had proved a difficult task for Sumi in Scotland, and for Maya and Indra, living rurally in the north of England and deep in Lancashire respectively. Many other nurses I interviewed felt lonely, understandably missing their families and friends back home. Until their family is able to join them, nurses try to stay in touch as much as possible.

Social cost of migration: family separation

Like Maya, Sumi, Kiran and Indra, almost all nurses had to make their first journey to the UK on their own, leaving all their kinfolk behind. Their solo journeys were of course made not by choice but because of work-permit, visa and immigration regulations. There is perforce a time lag between nurses' arrival in the UK and when their families join them here. The most common pattern of that journey has been traced in earlier chapters and only until some funds have been accumulated can they invite their families to join them. The UK Home Office's Border Control Agency requires proof of their ability to financially support their dependent family members. To arrive at this point seems to take nurses between two to three years on average.

Fifteen out of the 22 nurses I interviewed had migrated to the UK leaving their young children and husbands behind; three nurses were single and the remaining three came to be reunited with their husbands. During my initial fieldwork, I met nurses at various points on their journeys. Those with husbands and children in Nepal seemed to have missed their families greatly, but had remained in touch with them regularly. Sabita migrated to the UK leaving her husband behind, having been married for only a year. During our first meeting, she said:[5]

> I used to phone him and still do every day, I used so much money on the phone … it is hard to live like this, but we have no choice, I have to have a work permit visa first then I can invite him over, we are in the process now.

Usha had left her two children and husband behind and when I first met her, she was still looking for a full-time job. She explained:[6]

> I speak to them [her husband and two boys] regularly. I miss them so much, I tell my husband to look after them well and … *Mitho-Mitho Khanekura Dinus Bhanchhu* [I suggest him to give children tasty-tasty food or the food they like to eat]. Hopefully it won't be long before they could come here.

Like Usha. Sabita and Sumi, all the nurses lived in a transnational world, and those who had left their children behind were providing 'long distance mothering' care (Zimmerman et al. 2006; Parreñas 2005; Madianou 2012). Nurses constantly live between these two worlds: physically in Britain and emotionally trying to remain connected with loved ones in Nepal. These are some of the social costs migrant nurses have to pay. On many occasions, I felt all too close to home. Being a mother myself, when nurses started to share their grief at family separation and about how much they missed their children, it was almost too painful for me to listen.

I first interviewed Sabita in Scotland in the summer of 2007, when she was in the process of inviting her husband to join her. I had a telephone conversation with her in 2008, after her husband had joined her, and they were expecting their first baby early in 2009. In August of that year, I met a friend of hers and, on enquiring after mother and baby, learned that Sabita and her husband had taken their son to Nepal, leaving him there to be cared for by her parents. The reason for this, I was told, was because of childcare difficulties in Britain in the absence of extended family support networks.

Modern Internet technology has been very useful in helping nurses stay connected with families and friends in Nepal. During my time with them, I witnessed many nurses talking to their families, husbands, children and other relatives in Nepal. Sumi kept in touch with her friends in Nepal and internationally. She said:[7]

> My close friend is here. Now, here [in the UK] … the person who just phoned me a few minutes ago [she had received several phone calls during this interview], she is one of my best friends, from the hostel, my roommate [from nurse training time], some are here, one is in America, we do have regular chats, I don't miss them. But the people I miss are my parents and my *Dai* and *Didi* [elder brothers and sisters].

Many migrant nurses are able to chat via the Internet and some have discovered lower-cost rates on mobile phones.[8] Eventually, some of those dependent families who were left behind are reunited.

When Maya became more established, she invited her husband and two children to join her: the children started school and a few months later her husband found a part-time job in a co-operative supermarket in a village nearby. After the family arrived, Maya said she started eating regular meals with her family; she regained her health and put on some weight. She was happy, but her family did not like living in a rural village in Northumberland. A year later, her children felt that they had had enough of living in a rural area and wanted to move somewhere where there were other Nepalis. In late 2007 she began her search for another nursing post, contacting the same agent who had helped her find her first job. This time the agent offered her a few choices of nursing homes. One was in rural Oxfordshire, but in a location she felt was even more rural than her present situation. The next was in Callander, a small town in Scotland, with almost no public transport. Her children did not want to move there either, as they too thought it would be worse than where they were already. Finally, she found a nursing home job in West London, and moved there a few months after I had first interviewed her. I have met her several times since. So, within a year after the arrival of her family, she had to find another job, and all were uprooted to London. Some other married nurses have been through the similar pain of family separation, shared the joy of being reunited, and then had to adjust together to the different issues that relocation involves.

Family reunited: a dream comes true, but are dependent husbands happy here?

In addition to meeting with the nurses, I also met some nurses' husbands and children in the UK. After spending some time with the families, I learned that not all husbands were happy with their move and that some have found it very hard to adjust in their new environment.

Between 2006 and 2009, I met the husbands of 13 nurses: eight were husbands of the nurses I interviewed, and the remaining five men with whom I conversed I had met less formally. I have been in touch with some of these families regularly and have noticed some major challenges for these men with regard to the social adjustments they have had to make, resulting from changes in gender roles and traditional Nepali family dynamics. Generally, Nepali men are perceived as being the head of their household and the main breadwinner for the family. They take the main decision-making roles and the majority of men enjoy higher social positions than women. Their arrival in the UK as migrant nurses' dependent husbands, as their UK visa status suggests, challenges their family role and social position. Their wives had better job opportunities and earning potential in the UK, and quite often spoke better English. Moving to Britain means men have to make compromises in their social positions, sometimes giving up their respectable jobs in Nepal, only to find themselves undertaking undesirable, low-paid, and like Maya's husband (above), 'supermarket shelf-filling', kinds of jobs. Table 5.1 illustrates what nurses' husbands did in Nepal before their migration and what they were doing at the time of my meeting with them.

In addition to the above eight men, I met several other nurses' husbands in Hastings and other places, albeit very briefly.[9] Their wives informed me that, after arriving in the UK, some of them worked in restaurants in Hastings. After a period of intermittent joblessness and considerable frustration, some of them decided to join together and start their own Nepali restaurant business.[10] For some of the men, working in supermarkets as shelf-fillers, or in nursing homes as carers, was demoralising, and it was even harder to tell their friends in Nepal what kind of jobs they had been doing in the UK. Some of the nurses' husbands felt able, after a while, to share some of their frustrations about working and living in the UK, in informal conversations with me. I present two nurses' husbands' stories to illustrate how Nepali men have experienced their lives in Britain as dependent husbands, in compromised social positions.

I met Prakash (05 in Table 5.1) for the first time in spring 2007. He told me that before moving to the UK he was running a small but successful business in Kathmandu. When his wife expressed her desire to migrate, he agreed with her plan and fully supported her. They sold his business and used the money to pay the migration broker in Kathmandu. After a period of negotiation with this broker, they agreed to pay the top amount, which would guarantee his wife a work permit for four years. They wanted to have this guarantee after selling their business, so that she would not face any problems with finding a job in the UK.

Table 5.1 Nurses' husbands and their social/professional mobility after migration

ID number	Last job in Nepal	Job in the UK at the time of meeting (2007–2009)	Job in 2019
01	Senior government officer	Tesco shelf-filler	Tesco supermarket branch manager
02	Academic administrator	Security guard	Retired in 2016
03	Laboratory technician: permanent government position	Supermarket shelf-filler	Part-time support worker, planning for imminent retirement
04	Ran a private business	Carer in a nursing home	Part-time support staff in a primary school
05	Ran a private business	Security guard	Owner and manager of a private grocery shop in a Scottish town
06	High ranking social scientist/consultant	Carer in a nursing home	Further education – obtained a master's degree in international development from a British university in 2018, and is still working as a carer
07	INGO worker	Carer in a hospital	Healthcare support worker in an NHS hospital
08	Computer technician	Support staff in a nursing home	Carer/handyman in a nursing home

Source: Author's own field data

All went well and she migrated to the UK first, found a job and completed her adaptation training in a nursing home in Eastbourne. She found a full-time job and already had a work permit, worked hard, saved enough money and invited her husband and their six-year-old daughter to the UK. Prakash explained to me, however, that after his arrival here he had great difficulty in finding a suitable job. After all possibilities were exhausted, they left Eastbourne and moved to Scotland, hoping that it might be easier for him to settle up there. After spending the day with his wife and daughter, I was ready to return home. Prakash insisted that he would walk with me to the train station. As we walked, he revealed that he had been feeling desperately bored and frustrated, as he had no job: he had nothing to do and no social life. He said: 'I started drinking, I was just too bored and felt isolated, I did not realise how much I had been drinking every day, and when I realised, it made me feel bad.'

When his wife was at work, Prakash revealed that he would take care of their little daughter and do all the housework: routine work for women but not for men in Nepal. During my interview with his wife, Prakash cooked lunch for all of us.[11]

The next case study is of Deepak (06 in the table above), a well-respected professional with a master's degree in Sociology from Tribhuwan University, on completion of which he had joined an INGO in Nepal. Working for many years in the rural development sector, he had been involved in action research, worked abroad for the Japan International Cooperation Agency (JICA) as an international expert, had been involved in many key positions, and had earned a good salary in Nepal. His wife had worked in an INGO-run Hospital in Kathmandu valley. There was so much *Hawa* [wind] and *Halla* (noise, rumour) about nursing job opportunities abroad in 2004–2005 that, as Deepak summed it up, she was 'caught by this bug'. As she was not completely satisfied with the management structure at her work, she wanted to move to the UK and so started the migration process. She paid an agency £5,000 and came to England as an adaptation student. Over a year later she applied for a permanent position in a private nursing home. She saved some money and invited her husband to join her. He obtained a dependant's visa and arrived in England in January 2008. I met them for the first time in East Sussex, just a few months after his arrival, and on many occasions afterwards. He shared his feelings with me: [12]

> I get so stressed, there is no intellectual engagement in the village, nobody to talk to, and my wife has to go to work. I feel that I only use 1–2 per cent of my brain, and the skills and knowledge I had acquired in Nepal is useless here. Sometimes I feel that this will drive me mad, I need to get out of it. I cannot live like this for much longer.

Nurses' husbands who have been living as dependent husbands have had no choice but to accept unskilled jobs. Deepak and some others, as the table above illustrates, had highly respected jobs in Nepal, and for them nurse migration has brought only 'downward professional and social mobility' leading them into frustration and disappointment.[13] Women being the leaders of migration and men being the followers can threaten men's masculine identity (Adhikari 2013; Charsley 2008; Kingma 2006; Gallo 2006; George 2000).

In the summer of 2008, I met several Nepali men at a social gathering in Hastings. Some were friends I had known for many years and others the husbands of Nepali nurses who had recently arrived as dependent family members. During an informal conversation, one man made a comment and all the others laughed. I did not understand the joke at first, so I did not laugh, but they kept saying *Yo Raniko Desh Ho* ['this is the queen's country' or 'a country ruled by the queen', that is, a woman]. They had to explain this to me. To them it felt like they were living in a country, and now also in a household, headed by a woman. Men had to follow women's rules, as they were more powerful, perhaps just economically, than the men here. Although it appeared a light-hearted joke at the time, as later became more evident it was said ironically and reflected some bitterness. Nurses themselves have to face immense challenges and hurdles in their career before they are able to invite their husbands to join them, but when they arrive, there are other challenges to face, as their men do not seem to be happy either.

It is not just nurses and their husbands who feel social isolation and the frustration of inappropriate jobs, but young children who have just recently joined their mothers in the UK also seem to be facing difficulties. Binita had left her young son in Kathmandu with her family when she first came to the UK. A year and half later, she managed to invite her family to rural Oxfordshire, where her son started attending a local primary school. Binita said:[14]

> My son is eight now. He does not like it here. He has no friends, no outside life. In Nepal he had lots of friends and used to play outside with local children. This does not happen here. If somebody comes to play with him, they play for about 15 minutes then they go back home. My son does not like it here, and he wants to go back to Nepal.

It is evident that whole families have faced, and continue to face, many challenges in this new country.

Overall migration experiences

When we look back to where nurses' journeys began and see how far they have come within just a few years, it is quite clear they have negotiated many difficult hurdles and challenges. Nurses have moved on so far, and many have succeeded in being reunited with their families. Despite this, it not surprising that some still feel *trapped* by their circumstances in the UK.

'I am stuck in a dream-trap'

As we have seen, many nurses' initial migration 'dreams' and aspirations have proven unrealistic. Like others, Binita migrated to the UK with many expectations and much enthusiasm. After a couple of years, her 'dreams' and enthusiasm disappeared and she felt 'trapped' in a nursing home in rural Oxfordshire. She said:

> I used to be very enthusiastic about doing further study and advancing my professional career. Now all my desires and dreams have disappeared. I feel that I am in a trap. I can't move around as my children are here, it is not easy to shop around for jobs, and I can't just go back to Nepal either. When we are ready, and our children are settling better, we plan to go back to Nepal. I want to take them back, but now I feel that I am stuck in a trap.

This feeling of being 'trapped' was echoed in Moti's testimony, describing her life here as a cycle of never-ending difficulties and challenges.

Moti felt just like Sumi, Usha, Kiran and so many others that she was so close to getting a job and settling in the UK but that the future remained still so uncertain and the dream out of reach. This fear of the future and crippling uncertainty is not confined to this group of nurses, for I met and spoke with many nurses who migrated to the UK as NVQ students, and to adaptation students, all of whom shared very similar experiences. It is not surprising that some have described it as getting into a 'dream-trap'. As previous chapters have shown, these traps are related to nurses' own professional development aspirations, their families' expectations, and the desire to become successful.

Visa and work permit regulations driving nurses into casual types of nursing

As Usha's experience illustrated, nurses have found UK visa regulations becoming more and more difficult every year, and this has had a direct impact on their work opportunities in the UK. Until nurses secure work permits, they feel continuously stressed and increasingly vulnerable. The situation today has become almost impossible.

In 2008, any person with a student visa had to return home and reapply for a work permit from there. Moti, Kiran and many nurses who came to the UK with NVQ student visas, had to return to Kathmandu to do this, but they found it difficult to go back because they felt that there was no guarantee that they would get the work permit visa transferred. I interviewed one UK returnee in Kathmandu, who decided to give up on work permit visa transfer to her passport. As UK immigration policy became tighter, nurses' anxieties escalated correspondingly. For many years, nurses would rather continue to renew their student visas by enrolling on education courses and then engage in more casual types of nursing. I met Usha and many nurses in this situation, although not all nurses were willing to share the full details of their visa and work permit situations and their working hours, because it is such a sensitive topic.

According to student visa regulations in 2008, foreign students could work 20 hours in a week, therefore no employer would give them a full-time job contract. It would be very difficult for nurses to survive with such a small number of working hours and the resultant small earnings. They were forced by circumstances to take any hours they could. As time progressed, they started to alter this and increased their hours, usually ending up working casual hours. Much depended on how well they impressed their managers. Many nurses with student visas seemed to be working more than 20 hours a week. One nurse said that an adaptation nursing student would be permitted to work full-time hours (or over 20 hours a week), as work would be part of the training; but another said that no student would be allowed more than 20 hours a week. It was not clear to me under what kind of part-time work contracts nurses had, but many nurses I met were working as many hours as possible, usually more than 20 hours a week, and in more than one nursing home.

As discussed above, Usha emigrated to Britain in 2006 as an adaptation student. She completed her training in 2007 and received her NMC PIN. After becoming a fully registered nurse, she had difficulty in finding a full-time nursing post. Expressing her extreme frustration, she told me of how she had travelled to many parts of the UK for job interviews; to Ireland, Wales, Scotland and many places in England. She felt that her interviews seemed to go well but she just could not get a job, and suspected that it was due to the changes in work permit regulations. These changes make it difficult for a migrant nurse who has a student visa to get a full-time nursing post. Employers had become increasingly apprehensive about offering full-time and permanent positions to migrant nurses. Many employers were not prepared to apply for work permits. When they realised that the candidate required a work permit to work full-time as a nurse, they did not want to proceed further. This was exactly Usha's situation. Completely exhausted by her search for a job and with her student visa about to expire, she had to secure a new visa quickly. The easiest way of obtaining one was by enrolling on any course, such as an English language course in a private college or an IT course, or anything. She had employed both routes before.

In 2008, for this third time, Usha needed to renew her visa, but still had no secure job. She said she did not know on which course to enrol next, and how much to pay an agent to facilitate this. In the meantime she was working 50, 60 and 70 hours a week. The day I interviewed her, she had worked the night shift. During the day she visited a private college in London to enquire about possible courses in order to renew her student visa. I met her again in the evening, and she was working the next day from 8 a.m. until 8 p.m. and starting a night shift from 9 p.m., only an hour after the day shift finished. She said she had to do this in order to pay the fees and send some goods home for her children. As she had no full-time job and no security, she might not get any work from week to week. She had to take any shifts whenever she could get them, usually casual shifts.

I found many instances of this type of casual use of healthcare workers in the private health sector in the UK where Nepali nurses work. In whatever circumstances the nurses find themselves, they are not willing to return to Nepal, as they are still keen to achieve their goals of freedom of mobility, through securing Permanent Residency status and of becoming successful in their careers.

No going back without being a successful person first

One issue that the interviews revealed is the apparent loss of *Ijjat*. As earlier discussed the term used is *Be-ijjet* ['loss of face' or social honour]. It is a *Be-ijjet* to return to Nepal without some achievements, after investing so much family money, time and emotion. Nurses do want to return to Nepal with a sense of social pride emanating from the security of having a permanent job with a longer-term work permit visa or having obtained Permanent Residency status. Having been successful in securing a promoted post or advancing one's career, and having achieved one's higher education ambitions, are further causes for celebration and praise. Without any of these a return home could be regarded as failure.

Some nurses who had entered the UK as students had to return to Nepal to change their visa status. Even this visit had been difficult and *Ekdamai Lajlagne* (really and truly embarrassing) for them. When people asked why they had returned home, they felt that this lack of tangible achievement was only too apparent to their relatives and a source of extreme embarrassment.

Kiran returned to Nepal in 2007 to change her status from an NVQ student visa to that of a work permit holder. She said it took her a long time to sort this out. Staying with her family in Kathmandu, she had not been open about her UK visa situation, but people kept asking her the same question: 'How long you are here for and when are you going to go back to the UK?' She found this very hard to answer. She said:[15]

> *Ekdamai Lajlagne – Be-ijjet Hune* [it was really embarrassing] when people asked me what I was doing in Nepal, why I was there for so long. I told my immediate family about my problem with the visa but I could not tell anybody else. After that entire struggle to come to Britain, all that emotion and money investment, we need to achieve something before we go, at least NMC PIN and a permanent job. I could not even tell my grandmother. When I said that I was on my holiday, people said that people in the UK cannot afford to have over two months' holiday, so how did I get that time? It was very difficult to tell people what my problem was.

Even when migrant nurses really want to return home, they feel they have to wait in order to achieve something in the UK first. Sara, whom I met in rural Buckinghamshire, was desperate to return home, but could not do so just yet, she said:[16] 'When I finish my ONP I will go. I would like to go to Nepal first, like *Tufan* [high speed wind; storm, typhoon]! Other things will come after that.'

As she explained, a return home could only be made on completion of her training, so that she could take some positive news, some evidence of success, to share with her friends and family in Nepal.

When migrants to the West return to Nepal for a family visit and a holiday, they are received with an almost celebrity-style welcome. Percot (2006) observed, while interviewing nurses in India who had returned from the Gulf, that a nurse was treated as special by being served with a cup of tea by her mother-in-law. A simple action perhaps, but a daughter-in-law in an ordinary South Asian household, with no international migration and earning potential, would not receive the same service from her mother-in-law. Rupa, a Nepali nurse in the UK, told me of her friend's return from England to Nepal for a month's holiday. Her family and relatives arranged a massive welcome party for her, and when she went to her room after the party, her bed was covered with rose petals. These types of welcome are signs of the highest social respect. For Nepali nurses and their families, migration to the UK brings significant symbolic capital. Nurses and their families do not have to accumulate a large amount of money, as being in the UK is in itself a big success: it gives migrants' families, friends and relatives much *Ijjet* and enhances their social status.

When nurses do settle in the UK, after securing their jobs and work permits, and once joined by their families, they begin to buy houses or flats and other commodities, such as cars. They develop and join new social networks in the diaspora.

Emergence of support networks

Nepalese Nurses Association in the UK (NNA-UK)

In 2007, when I met nurses, and in some cases their families too, a number of them expressed their interest in setting up a Nepali nurses' professional support network. Via their personal contacts, and mainly by word of mouth, they invited Nepali nurses across the UK to join them. The number of interested candidates expanded and, after completing some basic work, a group of nurses, led by one of my research informants, set up a Nepalese Nurses Association-UK in London in August 2008. The nurse leaders are based in London and organise cultural events, offering refreshments, and organising fundraising charity dinners charging a nominal fee (see Figure 5.1).

Nepali New Year is celebrated in April and *Teej* (a major Hindu women's festival) later in the year. These and other charity fund-raising events are advertised on a Nepali Diaspora website called 'Big Nepal'.[17]

Most importantly, the main idea behind establishing this organisation was to create first a support network and then perhaps to develop a trade union and welfare organisation for Nepali nurses. They now have annual general meetings and regular elections to choose the board to direct and lead the organisation. Today the organisation has grown much stronger and has been a major and positive influence on Nepali nurses' professional lives in the UK.

The NNA-UK made significant contributions to the healthcare system in Nepal after the major earthquake in 2015. Nurse leaders have been active in raising funds to build a birthing centre in Jumla district in Nepal. Nurses are also involved in various health camps, trying to reach hard-to-reach Nepalis in the diaspora, and offering them health education and screening for any ongoing health issues in the UK.

There is an emerging debate on the role of migrants in a diaspora contributing to the development and strengthening of healthcare system back in their home country. Despite much discussion, there is a lack of evidence on what role healthcare professionals in a diaspora, both collectively and individually, play in addressing the shortages in their country of origin (Devkota 2013; Wojczewski et al. 2015). Newspaper reports suggest that Nepali nurses, midwives and physicians regularly contribute to Nepal's healthcare system from abroad. As already alluded to, migrant doctors and nurses in the UK

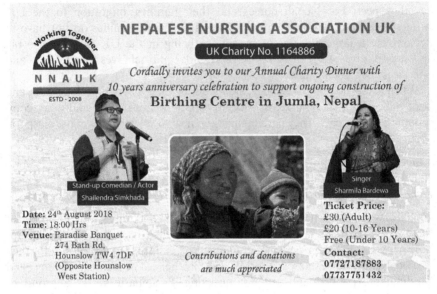

Figure 5.1 A flyer for the NNA-UK's charity fundraising event in London
Source: NNA-UK

contributed greatly to post-earthquake relief and health service provision in Nepal. There is a need therefore to explore the perceptions and roles of Nepali healthcare professionals in the diaspora, particularly their intentions to return or engage in circular migration and to invest, in order to ease the shortage of healthcare professionals at home.

Other diaspora networks

Similar to the nurses' network, various types of social support networks for the Nepali diaspora are developing in the UK. The total Nepali population, not just of nurses, is rising in the UK. The Runnymede Trust's research estimated that there could have been as many as 50,000 Nepalis living and working in the UK in 2008. That number had grown from 5,000 in 2001 (Sims 2008). But the Centre for Nepal Studies in the UK (CNSUK) estimated this number to be as high as 80,000 in 2008.[18] On its website CNSUK lists over 15 such network groups in London and Southeast England, of varying sizes. Almost two thirds of Nepalis in the UK live in this area.

Most networks of Nepali people were set up after 2000, although the Yeti Association was started in the 1960s, when there were very few Nepalis in Britain, and these were diplomats or came mainly from social elites. It remains very active in reuniting Nepalis.[19] In early 2019, Kaini speculates that there are over 500 Nepali Diaspora organisations to be found in the UK (Kaini 2019) (see Figure 5.2).

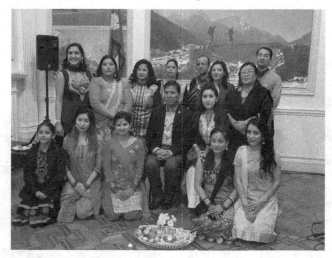

Figure 5.2 Nurses in the diaspora celebrating a Nepali festival at the Nepalese
    Embassy, London, August 2018
Source: NNA-UK

There is also a new network of Nepalis in Scotland called 'Nepal Scotland
Association' based in Edinburgh, with satellite groups in Aberdeen and
Glasgow.[20] There are some smaller religious groups, such as the Buddhist
Society, in London and new professional groups, such as the ex-Gurkhas
Association, and the Non-Resident Nepalese (NRN) group. Nurses interested in any of the groups, and who live nearby or within commutable distance, have joined these diaspora networks. These network groups also
organise and celebrate the major Nepali festivals of *Teej, Dasai* and *Tihar*
amongst others.

The growing use of Internet technology to stay connected with family and friends in Nepal and maintain socio-cultural rituals[21]

Skype and telephone facilities have been vital for maintaining family and
cultural ties while living in the UK. Chanda and Maheshwor, for example,
had a Skype and webcam assisted *Nawaran* (naming ceremony) and *Pasni*
(first rice-feeding ceremony) for their son (Figure 5.3).

According to Hindu religious practices, *Nawaran* takes place on the 11th
day after a baby's birth and *Pasni* at five to six months of age. On the 11th
day after the birth of Chanda and Maheshwor's baby, they held a *Nawaran*
very comparable to what would have happened if the family had been in
Nepal: three Brahmin *Pandits* and guests were invited to their family home in
Kathmandu and a few guests were invited to their flat in Edinburgh. For the
actual ceremony, a ritual *Mandap*, a temporary porch-like structure created
for worshipping and performing religious rituals, was established in their

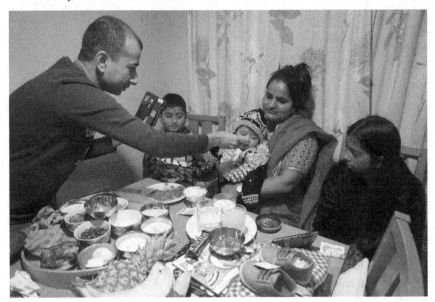

Figure 5.3 Chanda and Maheshwor's baby's first rice-feeding ceremony, Scotland,
        January 2017
Source: Chanda Adhikari

family home in Kathmandu and a *Pandit* conducted the rituals there. The
ceremony was planned this way because the family were aware that a *Pandit*
would not be available in Edinburgh.

At the Edinburgh end, the baby was put next to a webcam and was visible
to the *Pandits* on the computer screen, as needed for the ceremony. As they
performed the *Puja* (Hindu religious rites) in Nepal, they communicated
with Maheshwor and Chanda in Edinburgh. The *Pandits* read religious
verses in Sanskrit and gave instructions as to how to perform every step of
the rituals. The ceremony took a couple of hours, and Chanda and
Maheshwor followed their guidance meticulously. Everybody in the family
received *Tika*: a rice, yogurt and red vermillion mixture, applied to the
forehead as a blessing during religious or cultural ceremonies, or for good
luck, followed by feasting in both countries. Six months later, Chanda and
Maheshwor held their baby's feeding ceremony in a similar fashion, again
with a feast prepared for all the guests to celebrate. I was only able to join
them after the ceremony, but Chanda and Maheshwor had recorded it all on
their camcorder.

Chanda and Mahesh had their second child, Chirag, in 2016, and they held
very similar rituals for his *Nawaran*, and *Pasni*, such has become the norm in
the diaspora.

Future hopes

Permanent Residency (PR)

As we have seen, obtaining Permanent Residency status and a settlement visa in the UK has been a key priority and common goal, giving, as it does, nurses and their families greater freedom and mobility. Sumi's personal story in Chapter 4 illustrated this clearly, and the difficulty of attaining PR has been again explored as a theme in this chapter. I heard elements of Sumi's story during my interviews with many of the nurses working in the UK.

At the time of my initial fieldwork for this study, the UK Home Office's Border Control Agency regulation for foreign nationals was that, to become a permanent resident in the UK, a person had to live and work for five years as a work permit holder. After five years, she/he became eligible to apply for PR or a settlement visa. With this, a nurse no longer needed to obtain a work permit when she applied for a new NHS post or one in other areas: she could work wherever she liked. As permanent residents in the UK, nurses could obtain home student status, so would pay less in fees if they wished to go to university or pursue any further education course. They could travel to the UK and go whenever they liked, as long as they maintained some social links in the UK. For many nurses and their families, their main goal had been to wait for their PR. Nurses like Sumi, who had a permanent job with a work permit, were just waiting for this next step. This seemed to be another major achievement in their lives, one that many nurses were determined to obtain.

I met Kripa in London in summer 2007, accompanied by her husband and ten-year-old son. She was working in a private nursing home there, and waiting patiently for the time when she could become a permanent UK resident. She said: [22]

> Once we have the PR visa we can come and go in and out of Britain as and when we like. We have struggled so much and have come this far; next I just have to wait until I get PR.

Gaining one's 'PR' not only provides great relief and opens up many opportunities for migrant nurses, but it also seems to carry a huge symbolic value in migrants' social lives. It becomes the main success indicator and nurses seemed proud to be able to share this with their friends and families. When a nurse becomes eligible for a PR visa, and when she receives this status, it becomes public knowledge quite quickly amongst the Nepali nurse community. For example, in the spring of 2009 I was speaking on the phone with a Nepali nurse in Hastings. The first and most important piece of news she wanted to share with me was how many nurses she and I knew who had received PR in the recent months. She also stressed that PR is a major achievement for nurses, representing the new social status they have earned.

Being able to come and go as and when they liked gave them freedom of movement, and having choices about where they wanted to live and work seemed wonderful: a dream realised.

Desire to work in the NHS

Obtaining employment in the NHS seemed to be the next step for many nurses who were not yet in the system, and for those who had not given up hope. Access to an NHS job appeared to be as difficult as gaining entry into the UK for nurses from countries on the banned recruitment list. With PR status many nurses could step into the NHS, no longer needing to rely on their work permit or turn to agents for help. Nineteen out of the 22 nurses I interviewed initially said that this was their plan: to wait for a PR visa and then join the NHS.

Further studies

As illustrated throughout the discussion above, being able to obtain higher education in a British university is a major migration dream for most nurses. All of the informants said they would like to further their academic and professional specialist education. Some nurses wanted to undertake higher university degrees, as Sumi's story illustrates; others wanted to become specialist nurses. At the same time, nurses were aware that university fees would be very expensive, given that without a PR visa they were ineligible for home student status. Those who aspired to become specialist nurses realised that training places were reserved for nurses already working in the specialist areas, usually within the NHS. It was another 'dream' for them, and this desire to work in an NHS hospital had become their 'trap'.

Onward migration to the USA or to Australia

I met some unmarried nurses, who had more freedom to go anywhere they wished, and were frustrated with working and living conditions in the UK. They spoke of perhaps looking for other opportunities elsewhere, having found the hurdles of NMC registration and securing a permanent nursing job too difficult. One of my informants moved to Australia in summer 2009 and others were looking for opportunities in the USA. I found evidence of this on reviewing records in nursing colleges in Nepal. Letters of correspondence with nursing authorities in various countries showed some nurses were trying to move to the USA or to Australia while they were still based in the UK. Some nurses were preparing to sit the American Nursing Licensing exam from the UK. It is not only Nepali nurses, but also many other internationally educated nurses in the UK who are looking for better opportunities in other countries: this is now a widely known phenomenon (Buchan & Sochalski 2004).

Conclusion

This chapter has presented a mixed picture of nurses' social lives in the UK. On the one hand some nurses seemed to have very restricted social lives and faced many challenges in settling here. At the same time, there seemed to be growing Nepali Diaspora networks involved in charity work and fundraising activities to support good causes in Nepal. However, not all nurses have been able to utilise these networks fully because of time constraints, their geographical location and other circumstances. Wherever they were and whatever visa they held at the time, most of the nurses were waiting to achieve Permanent Residency status prior to working in the NHS. All felt that permanent residence would be the key to open up future opportunities: of working in the NHS and undertaking specialist professional training, perhaps even earning university degrees. Should they fail to do so, they would even consider moving to another country. However there would be no going back to Nepal without having achieved some success, be it the gaining of a higher education degree, the successful acquisition of permanent residence, or other, material achievements.

Nurse migration has created unsettling experiences for a period, not only for nurses but also for their immediate families, their dependent children and husbands in particular. All have faced the many challenges of social adjustment in the UK and have regularly felt extreme frustration at the quandaries in which they have found themselves. They are not yet ready to go back to Nepal, however, because it would be *Laglagne* or *Be-ijjethune* (a shameful or embarrassing experience) for them, and they would run the risk of losing face and of people in Nepal doubting their social position in the UK. As a consequence, achieving something tangible and visible remains very important for all of them. They must be seen as having successful professional and social lives before they could consider returning to Nepal, even for a family visit. From all my interactions with them it has become very clear that most nurses are trying to move to the UK permanently. On obtaining the historically, often only too elusive, full-time job and work permit, they can start to bring their families over here, buy a house, and invite their extended relatives to visit.

The final chapter will give an overview of this research, including the impact of nurse migration in Nepal and nurses' professional situation in the UK. It will conclude by discussing some policy issues on nursing workforce management.

Notes

1 Telephone conversation, March 2009.
2 Interviewed in East Sussex, England, March 2008,
3 Interviewed in rural Northumberland, England, May 2007.
4 Interviewed in Dundee, Scotland, June 2007.
5 Interviewed in Fife, Scotland, June 2007.

6 Interviewed in East Sussex, England, April 1008.
7 Interviewed in Dundee, Scotland, June 2007.
8 A detail discussion on how nurses and their families maintain family relationships and socio-cultural rituals while living in the UK can be found in Adhikari (2018), in Gellner and Hausner's (2018) *Global Nepalis.*
9 They were too busy to talk to me, so I do not know their professional background and they are not included in the table above.
10 When I visited Hastings and St Leonards-on-Sea, East Sussex in 2008, there were three Nepali restaurants, all having opened in 2007–2008.
11 It is unusual for a Nepali man to cook lunch while his wife is sitting and chatting with others in the sitting room.
12 Conversation with Deepak, Fife, Scotland, February 2009.
13 For a detailed discussion on husbands, please see Adhikari 2013.
14 Interviewed in rural Oxfordshire, England, February 2007.
15 Interviewed in East Sussex, England, February 2008.
16 Interviewed in Buckinghamshire, England, February 2007.
17 http://bignepal.com/forum/index.php?/topic/8319-nepalese-nurses-association-in-uk-cultural-programme, accessed on 4/9/2009.
18 Communication with the Director of the CNSUK, Edinburgh, Scotland, April 2009.
19 www.yetiuk.org/static.php?cate=About per cent20Us, accessed on 4/9/2009.
20 Further information is available online at: http://nepalscotland.org/index.php, accessed on 4/9/2009.
21 Please also see Adhikari (2018), Chapter 16; and Gellner and Hausner (2018).
22 Interviewed in London, England, March 2007.

6   Concluding discussion

Professional nursing in Nepal and nurse migration to the UK

Before closing this book, I revisit my original research questions: *why* do Nepali nurses migrate to the UK and *how* do they experience the whole process from their time as nurses in Nepal, through their migration journeys to their settling in the UK? I also summarise some of the major impacts international nurse migration has on professional nursing, and on the wider healthcare system in Nepal (as the source country) and in the UK (as the migrant receiving country). I consider this study to be not merely an academic exercise, but believe the findings are valuable in their potential to inform and influence nurse education and labour market policies. Ultimately I would hope that they might bring about greater workforce retention and improvements in health service provision both in Nepal and in the UK. I explore key policy issues, of importance to health service managers and policy makers in both countries. Given the current context of global nursing shortages, the unequal distribution of healthcare resources nationally and globally and, crucially, international nurse migration, particularly from low-income to affluent countries, these findings may be relevant to many other countries facing similar challenges.

We found international nurse migration, particularly from low-income countries, to be a highly gendered phenomenon, and to be an almost exclusively 'female only' issue in Nepal. Migration opportunities for Nepali nurses, the very first generation of professional women who travelled to the UK (and to the USA and Australia), have contributed to a profound social transformation, at least in nurses' and their families' lives, with concomitant wider changes in gendered roles in Nepali society.

Driven principally by global health inequalities, many factors have contributed to what has been an exponential growth of international nurse migration. Globalisation in technology and the increased availability of cheaper, faster and more frequent travel have helped to accelerate the flow of international migration. Migrants have instant access to information via social media and the Internet, and through various diaspora networks in the UK. Immigration and professional licensing policies, and the job market in destination countries at the time, greatly affect how Nepali nurses experience their professional migration journey to the UK and elsewhere. As seen in earlier chapters, the NMC UK registration process, and the UK's immigration and work permit policies, have acted as barriers or control mechanisms for the migration of Nepali nurses. Despite this they have remained determined to try and follow their dreams, given the availability of nursing or care work in private nursing homes, and the availability of NVQ and health-related courses in further education colleges.

I conclude by reiterating my focus on the nursing workforce situation in Nepal, highlighting the impact of nurse migration on nurse education and the labour market situation, and on the wider society. I finally reflect on professional and social aspects of Nepali nurses' lives in the UK.

The impact of international nurse migration on nurse education, the nursing labour market and health service provision in Nepal

Although there is an increasing recognition that international nurse migration can have a major impact on nurse education, the nursing labour market and ultimately on health service provision in source countries, it is an area that has not been fully explored in the past (Matsuno 2008; Hancock 2008; Buchan 2008; Kingma 2006). Drawing on evidence from Nepal, this book fills this empirical gap.

As Chapter 1 shows, the nurse education system in Nepal has undergone a series of profound transformations, mainly since the 1990s: from nursing becoming an attractive female profession to privatisation in nurse education leading to a sharp rise in education capacity. From being a profession suitable, almost exclusively, for a small number of urban-educated and comparatively well-off families (in the 1950s and 1960s) to a profession attractive to vast number of emerging middle-class women from diverse socio-cultural and geographical backgrounds, in recent decades it has become even more accessible for a wider population.

Unfortunately, the rapid expansion in education capacity has lacked adequate preparation, provision of the necessary human and physical resources and, importantly, robust policy regulation. The production of this surplus workforce has resulted in training resources being completely overstretched. This grievous situation is compounded because many senior and experienced nurses, from a relatively small pool of key professionals, are migrating to the UK, USA and Australia. Nepal's nurse education system has already lost, and continues to lose, many highly qualified, talented and experienced academicians and practitioners. Disappointingly there has been very little effort made by nurse education institutions to strengthen their own academic faculty and improve retention.

In addition, the nursing education curriculum in Nepal has been modified to match the nursing skills needed by the popular destination countries, mainly the UK and USA. New nursing programmes have been developed to meet international needs. Witness the new B.Sc. Nursing courses, begun in Nepal in the 2004–2005 academic session, but with no posts in Nepal created for B.Sc. nurse graduates. These changes have been justified as bringing Nepali nursing education up to 'international standards'. Such new developments have conspicuously ignored Nepal's domestic health service priorities.

As the World Health Organisation, and other authorities, have emphasised, international nurse migration from low-income countries such as Nepal has adverse effects on nursing service provision in the source countries, causing further inequality in health (WHO 2006). As increasing numbers of Nepali nurses are considering international opportunities, government-run hospitals, particularly those outside of the capital city Kathmandu, have been chronically understaffed, and this neglect has worsened annually (Adhikari 2014; NSI 2006; Justice 1984). As seen in Chapter 1, the recruitment, deployment and retention of nurses in rural hospitals and health facilities has been a major challenge for the MoHP.

Urban hospitals in Nepal face a different set of nursing workforce management challenges, as nursing staff turnover in most institutions is exceptionally fast. Tribhuwan University Teaching Hospital (TUTH) is one such example of this. One of the major state-funded teaching hospitals, and formerly viewed as one of the most desirable work places in Nepal, it is now severely affected by international nurse migration. In summer 2005, four ICU specialist nurses left TUTH in just one week. Clearly, it takes many years for TUTH to prepare a suitable workforce for these highly specialised units. In many instances, TUTH has sent nurses, and doctors, to Japan for advanced training in various specialist areas, having received substantial support from the Japanese Government as regards hospital building construction and workforce development. Nurses have also been seconded for specialist courses in India. The departure overseas of highly trained, highly skilled and experienced staff is a huge loss for Nepal's health system. TUTH did not have any major issue related to staff turnover and workforce recruitment retention until early 2000.

It is not only senior and experienced nurses who leave. Young and newly qualified nurses do not seem to be interested in establishing their future careers in Nepal. Their aspirations to leave are shaped by the broader culture of migration in Nepali society (Sharma 2018). As a result of the loss through migration of both young and talented, and of senior and experienced nurses, some feel that 'now in Nepal there are only elderly ladies left behind doing nursing' (Subedi 2006). The crucial question of what will happen when these 'elderly ladies' retire remains unanswered.

As already cited, TUTH is regarded as one of most desirable hospitals for nurses in which to work. This is in part due to its salary and other benefits, but even this prestigious institution has been finding difficulties in retaining nurses. In January 2018, the *Himalayan Times,* Nepal's national daily, reported on this very issue, revealing that over 200 nurses had left TUTH in the past three years: a significant loss of workforce out of a total of just under 600 nursing positions in the hospital. In recent years, nurses are being recruited every few months, reported the TUTH's Nursing Director (*Himalayan*

Times 2018; TUTH 2018). This type of unstable workforce has a profound impact on future workforce management, future planning, and ultimately on patients' safety and the quality of health service provision.

Lack of leadership at national policy level

International nurse migration has contributed to poor, or absent, nursing leadership development opportunities in Nepal. Chapter 1 has illustrated how the lamentable situation of an unregulated and exploitative nursing labour market has been exacerbated by a lack of nursing leadership in the MoHP, where the country's nursing policy decisions are made. Evidently, the migration of young talent and experienced professionals has taken the pressure off the leaders and policy makers, as regards their professional and political accountability. This ultimately impacts on the professional regulation, solidarity, and accountability imperative for a labour market. It is a market that should be seeking to be of the highest quality: attractive to applicants, effective, ethical and egalitarian.

Another crucial issue, identified by the current Chief Nursing Officer, is that there are only a few policy level positions for nurses to influence most professional nursing-related policies. This has been the situation for decades. During my initial research fieldwork (2006–2009) these higher positions became vacant, with the Chief Nursing Officer's post remaining unfilled for many years. Eventually the position was filled, but the new Chief Nursing Officer struggled to formulate better employment conditions for nurses, having received little cooperation from her MoHP colleagues, or from bureaucrats or medical counterparts at policy level. With such poor nursing leadership in workforce planning and with weak coordination and joint planning between nurse educating and nurse employing authorities, the situation has become critical. Such major concerns for the health system need immediate attention.

Commoditisation and commercialisation of nursing and the healthcare profession: increased private sector involvement

The political economy of international nurse migration has been a key thread running throughout this book. We discussed in full the issue of privatisation in nursing education and the many satellite businesses that have emerged around international migration. Applicant numbers for nursing education increase annually, feeding the market conditions for a now burgeoning private sector involvement. Nursing, as with many other types of technical and professional education, is now seen as a commercial opportunity. Professional education is available for those who can afford to pay. It is notable that many middle-class parents begin channelling their daughters' education from their earliest years, enrolling them in private schools, so they are academically better prepared to secure a future place in the competitive recruitment process for nurse education. Many young nurses are therefore from economically advantaged sections of society. While there are young women from poorer socio-economic backgrounds, who would also consider nursing as a career, they stand no chance of being accepted if their parents are not able to meet the training costs, and as seen in Chapter1, nursing course fees are high. There are only a very few scholarships available for exceptionally talented students. Ironically, these talented individuals are also unlikely to remain in Nepal, as they too have greater career ambitions, and will seek international opportunities soon after graduation.

As identified in Chapter 1, another important issue, and one that continues to flourish, is that many Nepali politicians and business entrepreneurs have vested interests in the health sector, establishing large hospitals, medical colleges, nursing colleges or training institutions for other types of paramedic professionals. Money has been invested in some world-class medical facilities in the past decade. Grande International Hospital, Norvic International Hospital, Om Hospital, Global Hospital, Nobel Hospital, Medicare Hospital and numerous other large modern hospitals in the Kathmandu Valley and other major urban centres, are just a few examples. All operate on a for-profit basis, targeting affluent clients. As these hospital services are expensive they are therefore inaccessible for the vast majority of the general public.

Professional nursing in Nepal faces many other challenges today, and ongoing political interference in the healthcare market is one of them. Senior nurses and those in leadership positions within the NNC, the CTEVT and the Nursing Section in the MoHP meet with a great deal of political interference, with politicians making regular phone calls to manipulate regulation in their favour.

Nursing labour market vulnerability and Saram Soshan *(labour exploitation)*

As of 2019, the nursing labour market in Nepal has remained as volatile as it was in early 2000. Given the ever-burgeoning number of nurse education places, with no sign, as yet, of the education market stabilising, the country is currently producing more nurses than it has capacity to employ. Every year new nurse graduates join the ever-expanding pool of unemployed or under-employed nursing personnel. Health sector employers in urban centres consequently have no shortage of candidates, so they can afford to use tougher selection criteria to fill any vacancy. New graduates find there is very stiff competition for posts, and it has become a new norm for them to work as volunteers for many months, or sometimes years, as a route into the labour market, before securing a short-term contract and then a permanent position (Adhikari 2014). Employers can operate under exploitative terms and conditions with impunity. With new recruits always looking for better opportunities there is no stability or long-term staff retention. Nurses' *Saram Soshan* (or labour exploitation), particularly in the private sector, is widely prevalent and has now become a prominent issue (*Himalayan Times* 2018).

Nursing being a highly skill-based and technical profession, nurses need to have an up-to-date knowledge base and to constantly hone and maintain their clinical skills. For all new graduates, it is better to practise their skills even under such exploitative conditions, than remain unemployed. Such *Saram Soshan* in the labour market has led nurses to continuously look for better opportunities, and fast staff turnover has become a norm. This pattern of poor long-term staff retention and the emergence of a volunteering system began in early 2000 and, despite much policy debate and activism toward fair pay and employment, the situation has not improved much as yet.

The numbers of private sector healthcare providers (in urban centres) are increasing fast, but there are insufficient posts being created to employ all new nurse graduates. As these private institutions can employ only a small number of nurses, it is often those who have better network and political connections (*Afno Manchhe*) who will be the ones to get jobs there. There is still no national employment regulation, no sustainable and fair employment policy, or indeed any genuine effort being made by employers to promote nursing staff retention.

In order to set national employment regulation and pay standards, nurses' activism continues to this day. The Nursing Association of Nepal, with support from the NNC and other labour-rights based organisations, continues to lobby for fair pay and for employment regulations to be in place: particularly the regulation of the currently exploitative labour market for nurses. In January 2018, and again in April and May 2019, an overwhelming number of nurses, from most health institutions across the country, came out on the streets to protest against *Saram Soshan* and demand fair pay for all nurses, and for the Government to take positive steps in setting national standards on employment, pay and other benefits. The problems of nurses have regularly became national headline news. The NNA was involved in mobilising those crowds of activist nurses. On both occasions, after several rounds of talks and negotiations with the representative of the MoHP, their issues were settled. However, under an already weak political system, with frequent changes of government (which is currently in the process of being restructured), these efforts have not been fully effective.

Since my initial fieldwork, the country has gone through further political transition, becoming a secular state in 2007 after a decade-long constitution-drafting and peace-building process. The country's whole political system was revamped, becoming a federal republic in 2015. It currently faces a new set of challenges, and there are plans to restructure its administrative systems and their governance, including the restructuring of the healthcare system. All of this has had a major impact on national health policy, service provision and on professional nursing education and the labour market.

Working in such precarious conditions, its not surprising that new graduates, as well as experienced Nepali nurses, continue to look for international opportunities. In 2015, a total of 5,916 nurses (about 15 per cent of the total membership) had formally migrated out of the country (NNC 2016).

As noted in Chapters 2 and 3, in the past decade Australia has experienced an influx of Nepali nurses. The number had reached over 1,000 by 2013 (Negin et al. 2013), and is likely to have doubled by 2019, as Australia remains a highly desirable destination.

Nepali men and women and nursing education abroad

Another significant development in recent years is that younger generations of Nepali men have started to choose nursing as a career, and in increasing numbers. Nepal did not offer nurse education for men until 2018, so younger Nepali men joined their female counterparts to travel abroad for nurse education, mainly to Australia. This emerging, and in recent years growing, phenomenon is difficult to quantify, as most graduates do not return to work in Nepal. Additionally, increasing numbers of nurse candidates travel to India to study nursing. As Nepali citizens do not require visas to live and study in India, it is almost impossible to estimate how many Nepalis obtain nursing qualifications from abroad, and where they work afterwards, and no study has so far been conducted on this.

Regarding Nepali students going to Australia for nursing education, anecdotal evidence suggests that young Nepalis enrol in a variety of other university courses, but some choose to transfer into nursing, as the nursing job market in Australia is perceived to offer better opportunities than other sectors. In the summer of 2018, as earlier related, an Australian nurse educator stated in her email to me:[1] 'I coordinate the Post Graduate module on "Reflection for Practice" and the majority (90 per cent+) of students enrolled in the subject are Nepalese.'

With Nepalis dominating student numbers, she sought what might be the best ways to support the educational needs of her students, even considering visiting Nepal to gain a basic socio-cultural understanding. I found this statistic difficult to comprehend but, as previously opined, given that UK-based Nepali nurses live in small clusters, this may also be the trend in Australia, and one such cluster may have decided to study this particular module together.

There are some positive shifts happening too: international migration opportunities for nurses have raised the profile of the profession. Recognising that Nepali men also have started travelling to Australia for nurse education, Nepal's nursing education sector has just decided to offer a total of 60 training places for men as from the academic year 2019–2020 (Tharu 2019; Khanal 2019). Most importantly, for some families, nurses and daughters are increasingly regarded as major family assets, no longer the family burden of the past, reflecting a broader change in Nepali society.

Nurse migration, contemporary social change and changes in gender dynamics in Nepal

An overview of professional nursing, and its relation to women's changing social position, has been highlighted earlier in this book. The professionalisation of nursing, and recent increases in attraction to the profession, reflect changes in women's position in Nepali society. For many women now are in paid employment, and indeed in professional positions.

Migration to the UK (and to Australia and North America) as symbolic capital: nursing and changing marriage patterns in Nepal

Nurses are viewed as desirable marriage partners for young educated Nepali men, and in general enjoy more freedom, independence and mobility than their predecessors. Thanks to gradual changes in the traditional practice of arranged marriage, a new generation of women now have a say when it comes to making marriage decisions. Only one generation ago, *Chhori Bigrye Nurse-le, Chhora Bigrye Commerce-le* was a popular saying in Nepal but, by the beginning of the twenty-first century, this attitude had completely changed. Now professional nurses are much in demand as wives, because their qualifications are not only seen as guaranteeing a job in Nepal, but also seen as a licence for the family to move abroad to affluent countries. Nurses have considerably more bargaining power, and gender relations are shifting. Since the advent of international nurse migration in Nepal, these issues are the frequent focus of media discussion.

An opportunity to migrate to the West has a great symbolic value in contemporary Nepali society, yet only a small number of privileged groups can materialise this aspiration. Money, an appropriate level of education, and the right social networks and connections are needed to realise the migration dream. Obtaining a visa to enter the UK, or any affluent country, in itself is already seen as a mark of considerable success in people's lives. To have social and family networks abroad, especially in the UK, the USA, Canada, Australia, New Zealand, or Japan, is viewed as a major asset for those who remain in Nepal. Seeing a family member make the journey raises others' hopes of migrating, or of starting a chain migration. The connections abroad and the receipt of foreign goods raise people's social status. People with family members, friends or relatives abroad are proud of this. This is particularly evident within middle-class social circles in Nepal.

By migrating to the UK, many nurses have enhanced further educational opportunities, not only for themselves, but for their children and even for their husbands. Most professionals in Nepal could never afford to send their children to the UK for schooling. Yet Nepali nurses' children are now at UK universities studying subjects such as medicine, business management and engineering. In Nepal, these professions are considered very prestigious, and indeed to be at the pinnacle of a career hierarchy. For these nurses' families, such opportunities would have been almost impossible if they had not left Nepal. This is yet another, and possibly the best measure of success for nurses and their families. At the same time, improved opportunities for women have made some men feel compromised socially. Men migrating to the UK as dependent husbands feel demoralised and frustrated. They do not enjoy the same social status they would have had in Nepal, and have little bargaining power in the UK job market. As explored in Chapter 5, nurse migration has had a profound effect on traditional male roles. For the Nepali Diaspora in the UK, not all men are the head of the family, nor are they the breadwinner (Adhikari 2013).

Finally, and most importantly, international nurse migration has created highly inflated expectations within Nepali society. Student nurses, newly qualified nurses and senior nurses, and their families, see nursing as a route to foreign jobs, as a sign of success and modernity that offers better futures for individuals and families. In following Nepali nurses' migration journeys to the UK it is clear that for some nurses their move to the UK has been a mixed blessing: often very painful, albeit eventually successful. Due to the considerable barriers nurses face, with tighter border control policies and more stringent professional regulation in the UK, not all aspirants can overcome all the practical hurdles and achieve their dreams. These unforeseen issues lead to frustration and feelings of failure when they find themselves stuck in their 'dream-trap'. Unfortunately, those still in Nepal, unable to obtain visas or lacking the right connections to even try to go abroad, feel that they are failures too.

Nepali nurses' experience and the contemporary nursing labour market in the UK

Deskilling and downward professional mobility

For several reasons, Nepali nurses have ended up in jobs in the UK that do not reflect their professional qualifications and experience, nor match their aspirations, and they have become increasingly deskilled. The complex NMC UK registration process has proved difficult to negotiate. The Department of Health in England's *Code of Practice for the International Recruitment of the Healthcare Professionals*' placing of Nepal on the banned list for active recruitment proved a further barrier. As has been cited several times, the subsequent UK Home Office policies and work permit regulations, designating nurses from the outside the EU as 'unfree labour' or un-free health professionals, was the final blow (Castle 2000).

The deskilling of professional migrants is a widely known and much-discussed issue. Many of my informants in the UK were highly experienced in CCU/ICU nursing, in theatre nursing, and in maternity services in Nepal.

After moving to the UK, and working in the care of the elderly and long-term care settings for some time, many nurses have lost their valuable clinical skills and experience, in management, teaching, and in their highly technical specialist fields, even though, paradoxically, some of these skills are highly sought-after by the NHS in the UK. Now nurses feel that they cannot even return to their former posts in Nepal, and they find very little opportunity for career progression in the UK. This is described by some Nepali nurses as a 'trap' in their 'dreams' and aspirations.

Professional class and un-free workforce

Migrants of various types are invited to fill vacancies for jobs, commonly known as the three Ds: dirty, dangerous and degrading (Castle 2000). These jobs are in the hard-to-fill category, and usually the least desired by the local workforce. Migrant nurses in the UK are faced with this same situation. Smith and Mackintosh (2007) argue that the present pattern of international nurse migration, and increasing commercialisation in the UK's healthcare system, has created a professional class; where a privileged, white, British workforce occupies the managerial level and the most sought-after positions, whilst migrant nurses increasingly provide front-line, hands-on care. Despite being highly qualified and having many years of work experience in various specialist and management positions, Nepali nurses in the UK are in the exact situation these authors describe, for the experience and qualifications acquired in Nepal are usually not recognised here. Many nurses are left with very little career choice, becoming tied to the work permit for private nursing homes. Compared to the facilities and privileges that their British and some European counterparts enjoy, Nepali nurses have certainly been treated like a second-class workforce in the UK's healthcare system.

Many migrants are tied to, or trapped in, their jobs. Castle (2000: 95–96) pertinently describes such migrants as 'un-free labour'. As Nepali nurses' situation illustrates, migrant nurses' work permits are attached to certain jobs in certain nursing homes; the work permit determines their professional scope. For the many who come from low-income countries, in trying to be an ethical recruiter, the NHS has effectively closed the door on them. Nurses cannot change their jobs or move anywhere easily, even if they feel discriminated against and exploited at work. Racism and bullying are perhaps most prevalent in private nursing homes, as illustrated through Chapters 3, 4 and 5, in the narratives of the nurses with whom I spoke. Mary's haunting story in the Introduction is a case of appalling exploitation. Eventually, vulnerable migrant nurses like Mary accept their circumstances, and discriminatory and exploitative practices become the social norm (Larsen 2007). The professional opportunities for migrant nurses shrink and they rapidly become deskilled.

No going back home, so no brain circulation

There has been considerable discussion in the literature around whether migrant skilled professionals, who return home with newly acquired skills, may benefit their society. This possibility has been termed 'brain circulation' (Kingma 2006). At the same time, there has been some concern about whether these new set of professional skills are at all appropriate in their home context (Mejia 1978; Kingma 2006; Yeates 2008). As regards Nepal, Nepali nurses would not return home with very relevant sets of newly acquired nursing skills. The majority of Nepali nurses in the UK are working in long-term care settings, and these skills are not so appropriate in the present healthcare context in Nepal. In addition, because nurses are becoming 'deskilled' in the UK, they find that they do not retain the same level of professional skills and confidence they had before migration, and so are not able to perform the tasks demanded in the posts in which they used to be so proficient.

Restrictive visa regulations have resulted in some nurses fearing that if they return to Nepal they might not be re-admitted to the UK. This fear keeps, or traps, nurses and other types of migrants, longer in the UK than they might otherwise have chosen to be. Thus these policies do the opposite of encouraging nurses to return to their own countries, where their skills are needed the most. Finding appropriate strategies to encourage and manage 'brain circulation' is important.

As indicated in Chapters 4 and 5, many nurses try to settle permanently in the UK, and indeed many have put down their roots, buying houses, cars and other commodities. Presently, most of the study participants have secured full-time jobs, and obtained permission to stay in the UK permanently. Many have their family, friends and relatives in the UK, and their children are in schools or universities. Nurses appeared to have settled here, so nurse migration from Nepal appears much more of a 'one way flow'. However, they do return home for family visits and holidays, and some have plans to retire eventually to Nepal.

The UK's healthcare labour market and the current context of international nurse recruitment

The UK has been experiencing a number of nursing workforce management challenges in recent decades, including 'ageing' or 'greying' itself (Dean 2009). There is therefore a valid reason to be concerned about the future supply of a nursing workforce in the UK. The NMC record for 2007–2008 showed that 31.04 per cent of nurses were aged 50 and over, compared to 27.3 per cent in 2003–2004 (NMC 2009). The total younger nursing workforce aged below 29 years fell from 10.46 per cent in 2003–2004 to 9.26 per cent in 2007–2008. When a large percentage of nurses, estimated to be over 200,000 out of a total 670,000, retire in the next ten to 15 or 20 years (Kendall-Raynor & Waters

2009), there may be a yawning workforce gap, which will need to be replaced somehow. It is not just that qualified and experienced nurses are greying or ageing, but in recent years more mature students have entered professional nurse education than previously, and these mature students have probably fewer working years than their younger peers. It would appear that younger people are not attracted to the nursing profession.

Additionally, from the late 1990s, in response to government efforts to increase nursing student numbers, there have been significant increases in those numbers: from 16,000 in 1994–1995 to 58,000 in 1999–2000. This enthusiasm, however, has not been consistent and sustained. Although the total intake has increased, not all students complete their training. The nursing student dropout rate remains consistently higher than average, at 25 per cent of total intakes across the UK. Even after completing their education, not all graduates register with the NMC to practise as nurses. The reason for the higher drop-out rate, during or after training, is believed to be the nature of job shift patterns and the higher percentage of students joining nursing in their 30s, a time when women usually start families and have other family commitments (Waters 2010). This high student dropout rate was estimated to have cost the NHS £57 million in 2006 and had risen to £98 million in 2008 (Waters 2010; BBC News 2008; BBC News 2006).

McGrath (2006) claims that even after qualifying, nurses are constantly in a 'should I stay or should I go?' state of mind. Some nurses choose to work part-time and others leave the profession early in their working lives, while others make international moves. For these reasons, the UK's health system has become heavily reliant on migrant health professionals.

The UK's nursing labour market, immigration policy and its overall international recruitment of nurses have been fluctuating, and still remain unstable, as of early 2019. In the last decade the international recruitment of nurses, as discussed earlier in this book, has continued to follow the pattern of 'turning the tap on and off' as and when needed. News of Nepali nurses being exploited, by IEC agents and also in private care homes in the UK, has filtered back to Nepal, so Nepali nurses' migration to the UK in the last decade has tailed off, and in recent years has become almost insignificant, with the migratory flow being diverted to Australia. However international recruitment, to 'patch up' nursing shortages in the UK, has continued.

It has been widely suggested that the shortage of nurses in the UK is due to poor investment in preparing the much-needed workforce, and poor workforce planning (RCN 2015; Buchan 2005: Stilwell et al. 2004). Despite regular alerts, and warnings of shortages in the UK, by the RCN and the Migration Advisory Committee, the Government has not been able to take an effective and proactive approach to workforce planning, before it hits national headlines and the situation becomes critical again (RCN 2017). The whole health workforce management process has been reactive to the labour market crisis, rather than proactive in health workforce planning.

Additionally, since the Brexit referendum of 2016, there have been further complications in the UK labour market. Brexit-related debate has dominated the UK political scene and has continued to do so. The past two years have been extremely unsettling for EU migrants already in the UK, escalating their potential vulnerability associated with job insecurity, uncertainty about citizenship and their legal rights to remain in the UK. Since the referendum there has been much political and media analysis and anecdotal reports of increased discrimination towards migrant workers and visible minorities living and working in the UK (Burnett 2017; Burnett 2016). Additionally, since then, there has been a 67 per cent increase in European nurses and midwives leaving the NMC register, with a significant reduction in those joining it, thus compounding workforce shortages (NMC 2018). It is therefore important that the reasons for leaving the UK are documented, and the experiences and views of this population are understood, and that any reports of racism and discrimination in the workplace are exposed and challenged.

Management of international nurse migration: discussing the key policy issues

International nurse migration is a complex global issue and so much is dependent on a country's economy and political system. For example, the NHS has been recruiting health workers from abroad since its inception in 1948. The inflow of this workforce began to decline in the 1970s, due to the global economic recession. This became even more evident after the rise in oil prices in 1973, which affected many countries globally (Buchan 2000). The recession pushed many countries into budget deficit situations, and healthcare systems in many countries, particularly low-income countries, were badly hit. The 1980s heralded a period of considerable global redesigning and restructuring of health policies, and other public services, not least the UK's NHS.

Slow global economic growth in the 1980s affected the UK economy, forcing the government to consider many changes in public funding. The Treasury was under immense pressure to reduce public spending, and the reduction in NHS funding was just a part of wider public service reform. Consequently, the total NHS workforce in clinical areas was significantly reduced. The cuts were to those personnel involved in direct patient care, such as nurses and midwives. By 1995, the total nursing and midwife workforce had shrunk to 343,380 from 397,030 in 1985, a reduction of 13 per cent, or over 53,000 nursing and midwife jobs in Britain (Buchan 2000).

Some of the Conservative government's policy changes and restructuring of the NHS in the 1980s were very unpopular amongst NHS staff, including nurses. When the Labour government came to power to 1997, claiming that it was inheriting a deteriorating NHS, it promised to make positive changes, and put more money into the NHS to improve the situation. Hospital waiting lists became high on political agendas and nursing 'staff shortages' in hospitals became headline news. The Labour government promised to deal with these issues quickly. This needed an injection of extra cash. Fortunately, a sudden economic boom in the UK helped the government find the extra financial resources to combat the long waiting lists and staff shortages. The Labour government promised to employ 20,000 more nurses by 2004, and in order to fulfil that promise the NHS needed to recruit more nurses and doctors quickly. The UK opened its doors to overseas nurses in the late 1990s, to address the acute nursing shortage as swiftly as possible.

After being criticised as an unethical recruiter, the Department of Health in England developed and introduced a *Code of Practice for the International Recruitment of the Healthcare Professionals* in 1999, which was further strengthened and finalised in 2004. The idea behind these guidelines, as already noted, was to stop or discourage nurses coming to the UK from low-income countries, including Nepal, and to support and strengthen those countries' vulnerable healthcare systems. Paradoxically, in some instances, some of these countries on the banned list have been facing significant health challenges and have been receiving UK aid to improve their own health services (Bueno de Mesquita & Gordon 2005: Stillwell et al. 2004). As discussed in Chapters 3 and 4, it did not reduce the number of Nepali nurses migrating to the UK.

If the UK is genuinely interested in strengthening Nepal's health system, it needs to focus on, and assist with, the country's specific human resource needs. There are several possible ways this could be achieved. The UK could proactively be assisting the Nepali government in making nursing an attractive profession in the country, by developing and implementing nursing workforce plans and retention strategies there, rather than by including Nepal on the list of countries from where nurse recruitment is seen to be unethical. Country-specific support and bilateral intervention is the pressing issue. An allocation of some of the money spent on the development of strategies and interventions by the Department for International Development, to support educational and career progression opportunities; improve health workers' practice environments; eliminate *Saram Shosan*; and ensure fair benefits and appropriate rewards in Nepal would be one step in the right direction.

The NMC and the RCN should take a proactive role to support migrant nurses in job matching

Nepali nurses, and migrant nurses from other countries, are already in the UK, and now is the time to use their valuable skills and experience, in ways that would be beneficial to both migrant nurses and to the British healthcare system. To make better use of these resources, it would help the situation if the NMC, the RCN and the RCM (Royal College of Midwives), collectively, were to take a much more proactive role, and adopt a fair and flexible approach towards the registration of internationally educated nurses and midwives to practice in the UK (Allan 2008). There needs to be greater control of the situation by the professional bodies. The UK's Border Control

Agency and private sector employers should not be the major players in dealing with such sensitive and important issues.

As explained, Nepali nurses have often migrated to the UK after acquiring many years of experience in maternity services and ICU/CCU and after having undergone specialist postgraduate training in Nepal. There was a shortage of about 5,000 midwives, and as many as 25,000 nurses, in the UK in 2009. The irony is that my informants (Maya, Moti and Usha) were highly skilled, advanced practitioners in maternity care and midwifery services, having undergone additional specialist training in Nepal. They have been gradually deskilled in the UK's healthcare system, trapped as they have been in the care home sector, whilst the UK continues to experience a shortage of this very workforce (Dean 2009; Duffin 2008). The professional bodies should together plan a learning support programme, and help experienced migrant nurses and midwives to move into their areas of expertise, and to achieve progress in their careers.

The need for clear and consistent border control policies in the UK

Although the border control issue was not central to this research when I started the fieldwork, it quickly became apparent that it is one of the most important issues for migrant nurses. It has a direct effect on the work permit conditions of nurses, and their professional scope and working lives, which subsequently determines their social and professional integration in the UK.

Some people in migrant-receiving societies such as the UK label those who come to their shores as 'economic migrants', travelling to the UK to siphon off the host country's national welfare and benefits. Although there is no evidence to support this argument, this has been the attitude of the governments of many affluent countries today (Winkelmann-Gleed 2006; Moses 2006; Moore 2006; Castle 2000; Hayter 2000). Stemming from this idea, most recipient nation states continue to create increasingly restrictive border control policies. But this seems to ignore nations' increasing interdependence, and the vital role of migration in keeping national economies active. Making border control regulations tighter than ever before encourages irregular migration, which keeps wages down, but it can also have negative consequences, as Massey et al. (2006: 13) states: 'As countries of destination adjust their policies in response to changing conditions, migrants adjust their strategies and tailor their schemes to fit the prevailing rules in regulations.'

This has been the case with Nepali nurses, as illustrated in Chapters 3, 4, and 5. The UK's changing of its border control policy, and Nepal being placed on the list of countries from where nurses are not to be recruited for the NHS, have impacted negatively on Nepali nurses, as they stopped being granted work permit visas. This did not mean, however, that Nepali nurses stopped migrating to the UK, as the NMC register shows. Nurses have found alternative routes in order to comply with the new regulations. They continued to migrate for some years, but with different types of entry visa. In short, the new visa and work permit regulations have not had their intended effect. Additionally, in recent years Nepali nurses have been diversifying their migration destinations, with more moving to Australia and the USA rather than the UK. The main intention of the DoH Code of Practice was to help retain health workers in low-income source countries. Clearly, however, it has had little or no effect at all on the migration of health workers from Nepal.

Encourage and support circular migration for brain circulation

Return migration refers to a permanent return home, and circular migration to a coming and going whenever desired. For circular migration, migrants need to have flexible options to come and go (Haour-Knipe & Davies 2008). I argue that migrants will return home, if they have the opportunity to move about more freely, and the option to return to their desired destination countries. This has been evident within the EU, where people had the freedom to move between EU member states after the 2008 global economic recession. The BBC World Service published migration data on 8 September 2009 which suggested that European migrants, in particular Polish migrants, were returning home (BBC News 2009). In a similar fashion, there can be thousands of Nepalis working in India at any time. Nepal and India have an open border policy. Nepali migrants go to India as seasonal workers, or some even spend many years there for education. After a certain period, some return home permanently and some continue to travel back and forth to India (Sharma 2018). This type of freedom is vital for return and circular migration.

Closing borders to professional migrants, particularly when there are skill shortages, clearly is not a remedy for the brain drain. Rather, bilateral discussions are needed to find dynamic and flexible solutions. In addition to this, modern day migration management could also include flexible professional exchange programmes. Many Nepali nurses expressed their hopes for greater freedom of mobility in their lives: freedom to choose jobs, to go to college and even to return to Nepal.

Unfortunately, as I have illustrated above, unlike EU migrants in the UK, or in other countries in the European community, migrants from outside the EU are 'trapped' by UK border control regulations. A more relaxed and flexible border control policy would greatly assist migrant nurses and other skilled professionals to return home. Such a situation would benefit individuals and the UK healthcare system. But when border control regulations are stringent, migration becomes more expensive and exploitative. Nurses become more vulnerable to exploitation by brokers and private sector employers, and to consequent 'back door recruitment' (Buchan et al. 2005).

The key importance of workforce planning and retention

There should be no shortcut and no patchwork solutions for the global nursing shortage: the only way forward is workforce planning and the promotion of retention. Nursing workforce planners, and international nurse migration experts, are urging all countries to pledge that they will prepare sufficient numbers of healthcare personnel for their domestic supply, and promote their retention to sustain that supply (Buchan 2005; Snow 2009; Kendall-Raynor & Waters 2009). Countries need to take workforce issues seriously and to be proactive. However, few governments have considered this issue seriously. Since the late 1990s, the UK has chosen short-term temporary solutions to healthcare workforce issues, following a path that effectively leads nowhere (Plotnikova 2012). It begins the cycle by declaring nursing a shortage profession and relaxing visa regulations for migrant nurses to be recruited internationally. Then the Government decides to increase domestic production (by increasing the training quota), and removes nursing as a shortage profession from the Home Office list, again tightening visa regulations. In a final turn of the wheel it stops all of these strategies for a few years when money is short, only to find itself back at the cliff-edge of a nursing shortage. This issue needs to be seriously considered. This is not just about projecting future workforce needs, but about financial planning, in which the role of external factors is crucial.

We live in a globalising and intensely interconnected world. External global factors impact enormously on national nursing labour markets. Education providers and employers worldwide need to consider these factors, and prepare properly to maintain a sustained nursing workforce. A Nepal-specific lesson is that education providers, as well as aspirant nurses, need to understand the dynamics and volatility of that global healthcare labour market. This research has shown that migration opportunities change frequently depending on the economy and workforce requirements of a destination country, and the global financial crisis of 2008 has more than clearly highlighted this point. The UK has seen a fluctuating workforce supply, with nurses leaving when they see better opportunities elsewhere. It is not only migrant nurses who leave, as seen in the NMC UK register, but UK-trained nurses have left for Australia in recent years. The current uncertainty around Brexit is another a very obvious example of an external factor that can impact on the nursing and midwifery workforce in the UK, and one that urgently needs to be considered (Buchan 2018; RCN 2017).

Government and society must value care work

It is the right time to explore and adapt ways to make nursing and caring professions indispensable globally. Nursing shortages and nurse migration are gender issues, and this book has highlighted the overall need to properly value nursing, and to see it as a highly important profession. Caring for the sick, and for frail people, should not just be seen as 'women's work'. Any healthcare system is a vital part of humanity, which should not be left to the private sector to create the sort of profit-making industries currently seen in Nepal and the UK.

Nursing is a highly gendered profession, and there is much exploitation of this workforce, in modern commercial markets in both Nepal and the UK. *Saram Soshan* (labour exploitation) is in fact a global concern. Gender pay gaps need to be addressed to create a fair and decent workplace for all nurses. There is a potential for the healthcare system, both in Nepal, the UK and globally, to benefit from an unemployed or under-employed health workforce, but this can only be achieved by taking a proactive approach. Valuing care work, investing in workforce development, promoting retention, and creating attractive working environments for nurses, can ultimately free vulnerable migrants, and all nurses, from the 'trap' of exploitative labour markets.

Note

1 Personal email communication, 4 June 2018.

Appendix

Brief chronology of professional nursing and midwifery in the context of the introduction of the bio-medical system in Nepal

1890   Bir Hospital was established by Bir Shamsher Rana in Kathmandu.

1928   The Rana government sent four young women (with their guardians) to India for 18 months of midwifery training. They returned to Kathmandu in 1930.

1933   The Civil Medical College was established in Bir Hospital, Kathmandu, training dressers and compounders.

1953   The United Mission to Nepal (UMN) was set up by foreign Christian missionaries to provide medical services in Nepal.

1954   The World Health Organisation sent two British nurses to Nepal to work with the Government of Nepal to establish a nurse training programme.

1956   His Majesty's Government, School of Nursing was established, first in Chhetrapati, and then later moving to Mahabouddha in Bir Hospital premises.

1958   The Nepal Nursing Council (NNC) was set up with the help of WHO nurse educators.

1959   Shanta Bhawan Hospital, School of Nursing was opened (under the UMN administration). It is currently Lalitpur Nursing Campus/Patan Academy School of Nursing and Midwifery (from 2016).

1962   The Trained Nurses Association of Nepal (TNAN) was officially registered, later renamed as the Nursing Association of Nepal (NAN).

1972   Nursing training programmes moved to Tribhuwan University (TU) Institute of Medicine (IOM), under the Ministry of Education. The Nepal Nursing Council was then dismantled, and training certificates were issued by TUIOM.

1979   The Bachelor's degree in Nursing, a two-year postgraduate programme, began in Maharajgunj Nursing Campus, Kathmandu.

1989   The Centre for Technical Education and Vocational Training (CTEVT) was established; undergraduate nursing programmes in the private sector were to be controlled by the CTEVT. It also initially supported ANM training programmes.

1995   Master's in nursing began at Maharajgunj Nursing Campus.

1996   The Nepal Nursing Council Act was passed by the Parliament of Nepal, and the professional regulatory body was re-established. A Bachelor's degree in Nursing began at Lalitpur Nursing Campus.

2009   Master's in nursing course offered at Lalitpur Nursing Campus.

2011   B.Sc. in nursing programme began at Lalitpur Nursing Campus

2012   Ph.D. in nursing began at Maharajgunj Nursing Campus: see www.iom.edu.np/?page_id=157, accessed on 20/2/19.

2018   Month-long agitation for decent pay and respect for the profession. Men (a total of 60, or 15 per cent of candidates, across the country in CTEVT affiliated colleges) are accepted for nursing education.

2019   Nurses out in the street again protesting against *Saram Soshan* and demanding greater regulation in training standards, quality and the labour situation.

Other global events that have impacted on nurse education and international migration in Nepal

1997–   The UK Government declared a workforce shortage and pledged to
1998   recruit 20,000 nurses over four years, to reduce waiting lists in the NHS, with consequent changes in visa regulation and work permit provision for internationally educated nurses.

1999   The DoH drafted a set of Ethical Guidelines for the NHS with regard to the recruitment of internationally educated nurses, particularly those from South Africa.

2000   A few Nepali nurses moved to the UK to work; slowly the number started to rise, and the flow was estimated to have peaked in 2004–2005.

2004   The DoH finalised the ethical guidelines for international nurse recruitment by the NHS.

2006   Changes in NMC registration policy: the Adaptation Course to Overseas Nurses Programme now demanded a higher requirement in English language competency. Increase in nursing education quota production in the UK.

2008   The Nepalese Nurses Association-UK was established as a charity organisation in the diaspora.
Global economic crisis: nursing was removed from the UK Home Office's list of shortage professions.

2010   WHO Code of Conduct released on ethical recruitment of healthcare professionals from international sources.

2016   The UK's Brexit referendum escalated anxiety amongst internationally educated healthcare professionals.

2019   Nursing skill shortages continue to be a political/policy issue in the NHS and the nursing labour market.

Bibliography

Acharya, S. (2006) *Belayatma Nepali nurseko bijog* [Pitiful situation of Nepali nurses in Britain]. Nepal Kantipur Publication Pvt. Ltd., Kathmandu.

Adhikari, R. (2018) Nepali nurse migration to the UK: transnational family ties, social ritual and the role of internet technology. In D.N. Gellner & S.L. Hausner (eds) *Global Nepalis: religion and culture in a new diaspora*. Oxford University Press, New Delhi.

Adhikari, R. (2014) Vacant hospitals and under-employed nurses: a qualitative study of the nursing workforce management situation in Nepal, *Journal of Health Policy and Planning*, available online at: http://heapol.oxfordjournals.org/content/early/2014/02/25/heapol.czu009.full?keytype=ref&ijkey=4pPQPh0duOyUUk6, accessed on 20/1/2018.

Adhikari, R. & K. Melia (2013) (Mis)management of migrant nurses in Britain: a sociological study, *Journal of Nursing Management*, special issue on nursing work, available online at: http://authorservices.wiley.com/bauthor/onlineLibraryTPS.asp?DOI=10.1111/jonm.12141&ArticleID=1173843, accessed on 20/1/2018.

Adhikari, R. (2013) Empowered wives and frustrated husbands: nursing, gender and migrant Nepali in the UK, *Journal of International Migration*, 51(6): 168–179, available online at: http://authorservices.wiley.com/bauthor/onlineLibraryTPS.asp?DOI=10.1111/imig.12107&ArticleID=1141134, accessed on 20/2/2018.

Adhikari, R. (2011) From aspiration to dream-trap: nurse education in Nepal and Nepali nurse migration to the UK. Unpublished Ph.D. thesis, University of Edinburgh, available online at: www.era.lib.ed.ac.uk/handle/1842/6199, accessed on 7/4/2019.

Adhikari, R. (2010) The 'dream-trap': brokering 'study abroad' and nurse migration from Nepal to the UK, *European Bulletin of Himalayan Research*, 35–36: 122–138.

Adhikari, R. (2008) 'The business nursing complex': understanding nursing training in Nepal, *Studies in Nepali History and Society*, 13(2): 297–324.

Adhikari, R.K. (2006) Privatisation in technical education: the case of education of health professionals in Nepal, *Regional Health Forum*, 10(1): 59–64.

Ahern, L.M. (2004) *Invitation to love: literacy, love letters and social change in Nepal*. Adarsh Books, New Delhi.

Ahmed, N. (2005) Women in between: the case of Bangladeshi women living in London. In KB. Tapan (ed.) *Transnational migration and the politics of identity*. Women and Migration in Asia, Volume 1, pp. 99–129. Sage, New Delhi.

Allan, H. (2008) Reforming (inter)national regulatory standards: the UK's failure to recognise and value the skills of overseas-trained nurses. In V. Tschudin & A.J. Davis (eds) *The globalisation of nursing*, pp. 103–115. Radcliffe Publishing, Abingdon.

Allan, H. & J.A. Larsen (2003) *We want respect: experiences of internationally recruited nurses in the UK*. Report submitted to the Royal College of Nursing, available online at: www.rcn.org.uk/data/assets/pdf_file/, accessed on 31/7/2010.

Baral, R. & S. Sapkota (2015) Factors influencing migration among Nepalese nurses, *Journal of Chitwan Medical College*, 5(12): 25–29.

BBC News (2009) Recession moves migration pattern, available online at: http://news.bbc.co.uk/1/hi/uk/8243225.stm, accessed on 31/7/2010.

BBC News (2008) Student rate dropout rate high, available online at: http://news.bbc.co.uk/1/hi/health/7337259.stm, accessed on 16/4/2009.

BBC News (2006) Many student nurses quit course, available online at: http://news.bbc.co.uk/1/hi/health/4711942.stm, accessed on 16/4/2009.

BBC News (2005) Concern over foreign nurse exodus, available online at: http://news.bbc.co.uk/1/hi/health/4556255.stm, accessed on 29/8/2010.

BBC News (2002) Concern over foreign nurse 'exploitation', available online at: http://news.bbc.co.uk/1/hi/health/1943820.stm, accessed on 29/8/2010.

Brewer, J.D. (2000) *Ethnography*. Open University Press, Buckingham.

Brusle, T. (2010) Nepalese migration: introduction, *European Bulletin of Himalayan Research*, 35–36: 16–23.

Buchan, J. (2018) We need a coherent approach to our NHS workforce woes. *The Health Foundation*, available online at: www.health.org.uk/blogs/we-need-a-coherent-approach-to-our-nhs-workforce-woes, accessed on 24/6/2019.

Buchan, J., B. McPake, K. Mensah, & G. Rae (2009) Does a code make a difference? Assessing the English Code of Practice on International Recruitment, *Human Resources for Health*. doi:10.1186/1478-4491-7-3, available at: www.human-resources-health.com/content/7/1/33, accessed on 15/7/2010.

Buchan, J. & I. Seccombe (2009) *Difficult times, difficult choices: the UK nursing labour market review 2009*, study report, available online at: www.rcn.org.uk/professional-development/publications/pub-003554, accessed on 20/6/2019.

Buchan, J. (2008) New opportunities: United Kingdom recruitment of Filipino nurses. In J. Connell (ed.) *International migration of health workers*, pp. 47–61. Routledge, New York.

Buchan, J., R. Jobanputra, P. Gough, & R. Hutt (2005) *Internationally recruited nurses in London: profile and implications for policy*. Kings Fund, London.

Buchan, J. & J. Sochalski (2004) The migration of nurses: trends and policies, *Bulletin of the World Health Organisation*, 82(8): 587–594.

Buchan, J., T. Parkin, & J. Sochalski (2003) *International nurse mobility: trends and policy implications*. World Health Organisation, Geneva.

Buchan, J. (2002) *International recruitment of nurses: United Kingdom case study*. Report, available online at: www.hrhresourcecenter.org/node/1195.html, accessed on 20/6/2019.

Buchan, J. (2000) Health sector reform and human resources: lessons from the United Kingdom, *Health Policy and Planning*, 15(3): 319–325.

Bueno de Mesquita, J. & M. Gordon (2005) *International migration of health workers: a human rights analysis*. Medact, London.

Burnett, J. (2017) Racial violence and the Brexit state, *Race and Class*. https://doi.org/10.1177/0306396816686283.

Burnett, J. (2016) *Racial violence and the Brexit state.* Institute of Race Relations report, available online at: www.irr.org.uk/app/uploads/2016/11/Racial-violence-and-the-Brexit-state-final.pdf, accessed on 18/6/2019.

Buse, K., N. Mays, & G. Walt (2005) *Making health policy.* Open University Press, Buckingham.

Cangiano, A., I. Shutes, S. Spencer, & G. Leeson (2009) *Migrant care workers in ageing societies: research findings in the United Kingdom Report,* COMPAS, Oxford, available online at: http://doc.ukdataservice.ac.uk/doc/6920/mrdoc/pdf/6920report.pdf, accessed on 21/4/2019.

Carlos, R. (2012) *The Filipinos' culture of multi-step migration and their retention as careworkers in Japan.* Panelist, Symposium 3, Migration of People and Intercultural Studies, Ryukoku University, Kyoto, Japan.

Castle, S. (2000) *Ethnicity and globalisation: from migrant worker to transnational citizen.* Sage, London.

Charsley, K. (2008) Vulnerable brides and transnational *ghar damad*: gender, risk and 'adjustment' amongst Pakistani marriage migrants to Britain. In R. Palriwala & P. Uberoi (eds) *Marriage, migration and gender: women and migration in Asia,* Volume 5, pp. 261–285. Sage, New Delhi.

Choy, C. (2003) *Empire of care: nursing and migration in Filipino American history.* Duke University Press, Durham, NC.

Connell, J. (2008) *The international migration of health workers.* Routledge, New York.

Cooley, D. (1982) *Shanta Bhawan – Palace of Peace: the story of a hospital in Kathmandu, Nepal.* Report retrieved from UNM Archives, file number 5–01.01.01.01.

Dalphinis, J. (2007) Discrimination in the NHS is rooted in exclusion going back hundreds of years, *Nursing Times,* 103(16): 12.

Dean, E. (2009) Investment, recruitment and support: initiative to tackle the midwifery crisis: analysis, *Nursing Standard,* 24(11): 12–13.

Devkota, A., B. Devkota, J. Ghimire, R.K. Mahato, R.P. Gupta, & A. Hada (2013) Involving diaspora and expatriates as human resources in the health sector in Nepal, *Journal of Nepal Health Research Council,* 11(24): 119–125.

DoH (UK Department of Health) (2004) *Code of practice for the international recruitment of healthcare professionals,* available online at: www.dh.gov.uk/en/Publicationsandstatistics/Publications/PublicationsPolicyAndGuidance/DH_4097730, accessed on 23/8/2010.

DoH (2001) *Code of practice for NHS employers involved in international recruitment of health care professionals.* Department of Health, London.

DoH (1999) *Guidance on international recruitment.* Department of Health, London.

Diallo, K. (2004) Data on the migration of health-care workers: sources, uses and challenges, *Bulletin of the World Health Organisation,* 82(8): 601–607.

Dicicco-Bloom, B. (2004) The racial and gendered experiences of immigrant nurses from Kerala, India, *Journal of Transcultural Nursing,* 15(1): 26–33.

Dixit, H. (2005) *Nepal's quest for health.* Educational Publishing House, Kathmandu.

Duffin, C. (2008) NHS could face shortfall of 25,000 nurses, *Nursing Standard,* 23 (4): 6.

Ehrenreich, B. & A. Russell-Hochschild (eds) (2002) *Global women: nannies, maids and sex workers in the new economy.* Granta Books, London.

Gautam, T.R. (2008) Migration and the problem of old age people in Nepal, *Dhaulagiri Journal of Sociology and Anthropology,* 2: 145–162.

Gallo, E. (2006) 'Italy is not a good place for men': narratives of places, marriage and masculinity among Malayali migrants, *Global Networks*, 6(4): 357–372.

Gellner, D.N. and S.L. Hausner (eds) (2018) *Global Nepalis: religion, culture, and community in a new and old diaspora*. Oxford University Press, New Delhi.

Gellner, D.N. & E. Hirsch (2001) *Inside organisations: anthropologists at work*. Berg, Oxford and New York.

George, S. (2000) 'Dirty nurses' and 'men who play': gender and class in transnational migration. In Michael Buraway (ed.) *Global ethnography: forces, connections and imaginations in a post modern world*, pp. 144–174. University of California Press, Berkeley, CA.

Ghimire, L. (2007) *BideshMa Basne Chhoraharu Narse Buhari Khojna Anurod Garchhan* [Sons who live in foreign countries request their parents to search for nurse daughter-in-law], *Kantipur Daily*, Kosheli Ka 12 sawan 2064 (28 July).

Hamal-Gurung, S. (2015) *Nepali migrant women: resistance and survival in America*. Syracuse University Press, Syracuse, NY.

Hancock, P.K. (2008) Nurse migration: the effect on nursing education, *International Nursing Review*, 55(3): 258–264.

Handwerker, W.P. (2001) *Quick ethnography*. Altamira Press, Walnut Creek, CA.

Haour-Knipe, M. & A. Davies (2008) *Return migration of nurses*. International Centre on Nurse Migration, Philadelphia, PA, available online at: www.intlnursemigration. org/assets/pdfs/return%20migration%20ltr.pdf, accessed on 9/8/2010.

Harris, D., J. Wales, H. Jones, & T. Rana, with R.L. Chitrakar (2013) *Human resources for health in Nepal: politics of access in remote areas*. ODI, Shaping Policy for Development, available online at: www.od.org/publications/7375-human-resources-health-nepal-politics-access-remote-areas, accessed on 20/6/2019.

Harper, I. (2009) Mediating therapeutic uncertainty: a mission hospital in Nepal. In M. Harrison, M. Jones, & H. Sweet (eds) *From western medicine to global medicine, the hospital beyond the West*, pp. 303–329. Orient Black Swan Private Ltd, New Delhi.

Harper, I. (2003) Mission, magic and medicalisation: an anthropological study into public health in contemporary Nepal. Ph.D thesis submitted to the School of Oriental and African Studies, University of London.

Hayter, T. (2000) *Open borders: the case against immigration controls*. Pluto Press, London.

Henry, L. (2008) Disengagement and demoralisation: the roots of Ghanaian nurses' responses to discrimination in the (UK) NHS. In V. Tschudin & A.J. Davis (eds) *The globalisation of nursing*, pp. 116–128. Radcliffe Publishing, Abingdon.

Herdman, EA. (2004) Globalization, internationalization and nursing, *Nursing and Health Science*, 6: 237–238.

Himal News Service (2007) Accord for placements for nurses in the UK, *Himalayan Times*, available online at: www.thehimalayantimes.com/fullstory.asp?filename=aNPata0sdqzp ca8Wa9ta.axamal&folder=aNPataiaoanaaal&Name=National&sImageFileName=&dt SiteDate=20080726, accessed on 17/1/2009.

Justice, J. (1986) *Policies, plans and people: culture and health development in Nepal*. University of California Press, Berkeley, CA.

Kaini, B.K. (2019) *Belayatma Nepali Sangha Sansthaharu, Kasto Chha Halat?* [Nepali organisations in Britain: what is the situation?] *Online Khabar*, available at: www.onlinekhabar.com/2019/01/738467?fbclid=IwAR3eZb1nmQeB_Ng862rm VScORWGuzaQlUNNRZn09iL2NR-S5lvn17DZYitc, accessed on 26/4/2019.

KC, S. (2004) *Pratichhayama chhan British ra American Aspatalharu* [British and American hospitals are waiting], *Himal Khabarpatrika*, Asar (June–July): 16–31.

Kendall-Raynor, P. & A. Waters (2009) Job cuts and ageing workforce spell nurse shortage timebomb, *Nursing Standard*, 23(30): 6.

Khadria, B. (2007) International Nurse Recruitment in India, *Health Service Research*, 42(3): part 11, Health Research and Education Trust, available online at: www.ncbi. nlm.nih.gov/pmc/articles/PMC1955375/pdf/hesr0042-1429.pdf, accessed on 30/6/ 2010.

Khanal, K. (2019) Nepal's nursing colleges reserve spots for male students, *Global Press Journal*, available online at: https://globalpressjournal.com/asia/nepal/nepals-nursing-colleges-reserve-spots-male-students/, accessed on 27/4/2019.

Kingma, M. (2006) *Nurses on the move: migration and global health care economy.* ILR Press of Cornell University Press, Ithaca, NY and London.

Kline, R. (2014) *The 'snowy white peaks' of the NHS: a survey of discrimination in governance and leadership and the potential impact on patient care in London and England.* Middlesex University's Research Repository, available online: www.england.nhs.uk/wp-content/uploads/2014/08/edc7-0514.pdf, accessed on 24/6/2019.

Kupfer, L., K. Hofman, R. Jarawan, J. McDermott, & K. Bridbord (2004) Strategies to discourage brain drain, *Bulletin of the World Health Organization*, 82(8): 616–623.

Larsen, J.A. (2007) Embodiment of discrimination and overseas nurses' career progression, *Journal of Clinical Nursing*, 2187–2195, available online at: http://online library.wiley.com/doi/10.1111/j.1365-2702.2007.02017.x/full, accessed on 12/8/2010.

Liechty, M. (2003) *Suitably modern: making middle-class culture in a new consumer society.* Princeton University Press, Princeton, NJ and Oxford.

Liechty, M. (1997) Selective exclusion: foreigners, foreign goods, and foreignness in modern Nepali history, *Studies in Nepali History and Society*, 2(1): 5–68.

Lindell, J. (1997) *Nepal and the Gospel of God.* United Mission to Nepal and Pilgrims Book House, Kathmandu.

Madianou, M. (2012) Migration and the accentuated ambivalence of motherhood: the role of ICTs in Filipino transnational families, *Global Networks*, 12(3): 277–295.

Marasini, BR. (2003) *Human resources for health development policy in Nepal: health policy analysis.* Unpublished report submitted to the Nepal Health Research Council, Kathmandu.

Massey, D.S., J. Arango, G. Hugo, A. Kouaouci, A. Pellegrino, & J. Edward Taylor (2006) *Worlds in motion: understanding international migration at the end of the millennium.* Clarendon Press, Oxford.

Matsuno, A. (2008) Nurse migration: the Asian perspective. ILO/EU Asian Programme on the Governance of Labour Migration, technical note, available online at: http://psta lker.com/ilo/resources/Technical%20Note%20-%20Nurse%20Migration%20by%20A% 20Matsuno.doc, accessed on 20/9/2009.

Maxwell, M. with R. Sinha (2004) *Nurses were needed at the top of the world: the first fifty years of professional nursing in Nepal 1951–2001.* TU Institute of Medicine, Lalitpur Nursing Campus.

McGrath, A. (2006) Should I stay or should I go? Towards an understanding of leaving nursing. Ph.D. thesis submitted to the University of Edinburgh, available online at: www.era.lib.ed.ac.uk/bitstream/1842/3178/1/McGrath%20A%20PhD%20thesis% 2006.pdf, accessed on 18/8/2010.

Mejia, A. (1978) Migration of physicians and nurses: a worldwide picture, *International Journal of Epidemiology*, 7(3): 207–215.

Melia, K. (1987) *Learning and working: the occupational socialisation of nurses.* Tavistock Publications, London.

Moore, S. (2006) Give us your best, your brightest: immigration policy benefits U.S. society despite increasing problems. In A.M. Messina & G. Lahav (eds) *The migration reader: exploring politics and policy*, pp. 329–333. Lynne Rienner, Boulder, CO and London.

Moses, J.W. (2006) *International migration: globalisation's last frontier.* Zed Books, London and New York.

Mosse, D. (2005) *Cultivating development: an ethnography of aid policy and practice.* Pluto Press, London.

NAN (Nursing Association of Nepal) (2002) *History of nursing in Nepal, 1890–2002.* Lazimpat, Kathmandu.

Negin, J., A. Rozea, B. Cloyd, & A.L.C. Martiniuk (2013) Foreign-born health workers in Australia: analysis of census data, *Human Resources for Health*, 11: 69, available online at: https://human-resources-health.biomedcentral.com/articles/10.1186/1478-4491-11-69, accessed on 20/3/2019.

Nepalnews.com (2009) US Embassy cautions visa applicants over fake documents, available online at: www.nepalnews.com/archive/2009/jan/jan24/news03, accessed on 13/8/2010.

NMC (Nursing and Midwifery Council) (2018) *NMC register*, 31 March, available online at: www.nmc-uk.org/, accessed on 20/4/2019.

NMC (2010) NMC approved programmes in the UK for nurses trained outside Europe, available online at: www.nmc-uk.org/Approved-Programmes/, accessed on 13/8/2010.

NMC (2009) Statistical analysis of the register – 1 April 2007 to 31 March 2008, available online at: www.nmc.org, accessed on 21/4/2009.

NMC (2008) Statistical analysis of the register – 1 April 2006 to 31 March 2007, available online at: www.nmc.org, accessed on 21/4/2009.

NNC (Nepal Nursing Council) (2019) *NNC Record*, available at: http://nnc.org.np/#, accessed on 29/5/2019.

NNC (2016) *NNC Record*, available at: http://nnc.org.np/#, accessed on 20/4/2019.

NNC (2006) *Nursing Sikchyan sanstha sthapana ra sanchalan ganra swikriti dine nikaya tatha nursing saitchik karyakram sanchalan garne sansthayalai Nepal Nursing Parisadko atayanta jaruri suchana* [NNC notice for those authorities who give permission to run nursing programme and the nursing institutes who run nursing progamme], *Kantipur Daily*, p. 8.

NSI (Nick Simon Institute) (2006) *Deployment of health workers in government district hospitals in Nepal.* Original research report, available online at: www.nsi.edu.np/nsi/research/3994HCW%20Report.pdf, accessed on 8/11/2009.

Parish, C. (2006) Overseas nurses stranded by lack of training places and placements, *Nursing Standard*, 20(33): 7.

Pariyar, G. (2005) *Syasthya ra Nursing: Aakarshak Kariyar* [Health and nursing: an attractive career], *Samaya*, Kartik 10 2063vs: 39–41.

Parreñas, R.S. (2005) *Children of global migration: transnational families and gendered woes.* Stanford University Press, Stanford, CA.

Percot, M. (2006) Indian nurses in the Gulf: from job opportunities to life strategies. In A. Agrawal (ed.) *Migrant women and work*, Women and Migration in Asia, Volume 4, pp. 155–176. Sage Publications, New Delhi.

Philogene, S. (2008) *Between two worlds: a narrative.* Author House.

Plotnikova, E.V. (2012) Cross-border mobility of health professionals: contesting patients' right to health, *Social Science and Medicine*, 74: 20–27, available online at: www.sciencedirect.com/science/article/pii/S0277953611000980, accessed on 29/5/2019.

Pollock, A.M. (2005) *NHS plc: the privatisation of our health care.* Verso, London.

Rai, M.K. (2009) *Nursing Shikshayama Satarka* [Be aware of nursing education], *Nagarik*, 10.

Rankin, K.N. (2004*) The cultural politics of markets: economic liberalisation and social change in Nepal.* Pluto Press, London.

RCN (Royal College of Nursing) (2017) Worst case scenario: shortage of 42,000 nurses: After Brexit the NHS could be hit by a shortage of nurses by 2026, available online at: www.rcn.org.uk/news-and-events/news/worst-case-scenario-shortage-of-42000-nurses, accessed on 20/6/2019.

RCN (2016) *Unheeded warnings: healthcare in crisis. The UK nursing labour market review 2016,* available online at: www.rcn.org.uk/professional-development/publications/pub-005779, accessed on 20/6/2019.

RCN (2015) *A workforce in crisis? The UK nursing labour market review 2015,* available online at: www.rcn.org.uk/professional-development/publications/pub-005348, accessed on 20/6/2019.

RCN (2007) *Black and minority ethnic and internally recruited nurses: results from RCN Employment/Working Well surveys 2005 and 2002,* available online at: www.rcn.org.uk/professional-development/publications/pub-003104, accessed on 20/6/2019.

RCN (2005) *Success with internationally recruited nurses: RCN good practice guidance for employers in recruiting and retaining,* available online at: www.rcn.org.uk/_data/assets/pdf_file/0010/78625/002445.pdf, accessed on 28/8/2010.

RCN (2003) *Here to stay? International nurses in the UK,* available online at: www.rcn.org.uk/__data/assets/pdf_file/0011/78563/001982.pdf, accessed on 28/8/2010.

Red Pepper (2004) *Modern heroes, modern slaves,* available online at: www.redpepper.org.uk/Modern-heroes-modern-slaves, accessed on 29/8/2010.

Ritchie, J. & J. Lewis (2003) *Qualitative research practice: a guide for social science students and researchers.* Sage, London.

Rozario, S. (2005) Singular predicaments: unmarried female migrants and the changing Bangladeshi family. In M. Thapan (ed.) *Transnational migration and the politics of identity: women and migration in Asia,* Volume 1, pp. 150–180. Sage Publications, New Delhi.

Saravia, N.G. & J.F. Miranda (2004) Plumbing the brain drain, *Bulletin of the World Health Organisation*, 82(8): 608–615.

Sassen, S. (2006) Global cities and survival circuits. In M.K. Zimmerman, J.S. Litt, & C.E. Bose (eds) *Global dimensions of gender and carework*, pp. 30–38. Stanford University Press, Stanford, CA.

Seddon, D., J. Adhikari, & G. Gurung (2001) *New lahure: foreign employment and remittance economy of Nepal.* Nepal Institute of Development Studies, Kathmandu.

Shakya, S. (2009) *Unleashing Nepal: past, present and the future of the economy.* Penguin Books, New Delhi.

Sharma, J.R. (2018) *Crossing the border to India: youth, migration and masculinities in Nepal.* Temple University Press, Philadelphia PA.

Shelley, T. (2007) *Exploited: migrant labour in the new global economy*. Zed Books, London and New York.

Sims, JM. (2008) *Soldiers, migrants and citizens: the Nepalese in Britain*. A Runnymede Trust Community Study, available online at: www.runnymedetrust.org/uploads/publications/pdfs/TheNepaleseInBritain-2008.pdf, accessed on 30/8/2010.

Smith, P. & M. Mackintosh (2007) Profession, market and class: nurse migration and remaking of division and disadvantage, *Journal of Clinical Nursing*, 2213–2220.

Smith, P., H. Allan, L. Henry, J. Larsen, & M. Mackintosh (2006) *Valuing and recognising the talents of a diverse healthcare workforce: report from the REOH study: researching equal opportunities for overseas-trained nurses and other healthcare professionals*. European Union, Royal College of Nursing, University of Surrey and the Open University, available online at: www.rcn.org.uk/_data/assets/pdf_file/0008/78713/003078.pdf, accessed on 8/8/2010.

Snow, T. (2009) Workforce planning tops agenda to prevent shortfall of nurses, *Nursing Standard*, 24(3): 12–13.

Spitzer, D., A. Neufeld, M. Harrison, K. Hughes, & M. Stewart (2006) Caregiving in transnational context: 'my wings have been cut; where can I fly?' In M.K. Zimmerman, J.S. Litt, & C.E. Bose (eds) *Global dimensions of gender and carework*, pp. 176–188. Stanford University Press, Stanford, CA.

Stilwell, B., K. Diallo, P. Zurn, M. Vujicic, O. Adams, & M. Dal Poz (2004) Migration of health-care workers from developing countries: strategic approaches to its management, *Bulletin of the World Health Organisation*, 82(8): 595–600, available online at: www.who.int/workforcealliance/11.pdf, accessed, on 20/6/2019.

Subba, A. (2008) Power of correct info. *Himalayan Times*, 11 November, p. 13.

Subedi, A. (2006) Nurses flock abroad though badly needed here, available at: http://Kantipuronline.com/kolnews.php?&nid=95901, accessed on 21/1/2009.

Subedi, M.S. (2001) *Medical anthropology of Nepal*. Udaya Books, Kathmandu.

SWiFT (Study on Work in Freedom Transnational – Evaluation) (2017) Transnational female labour migration: perspective of low-wage Nepalese workers, Nepal briefing note, emerging findings from SWiFT evaluation, available online at: http://same.lshtm.ac.uk/files/2018/02/SWIFT_-Nepal-briefing-note-03-Dec2017-V2.pdf, accessed on 5/5/2019.

Thakur, L. (1999) Training of professional nurses in Nepal, *Journal of the Institute of Medicine*, 21: 110–115.

Thapa, B. (2009) *Chhori sapriya 'nursele'* [A daughter is improved by becoming a 'nurse'], *Kantipur*, 5 September (19th bhadau 2066 vs).

Thapan, M. (2005) *Transnational migration and politics of identity, women and migration in Asia*, Volume 1. Sage Publications, New Delhi.

Tharu, B. (2019) Nepalma 60 jana purus Narsing Padhai chha! Kun College ma Kati? [In Nepal, 60 men are studying nursing! How many in which college?], *Swasthaya Khabar Patrika*, available online at: https://Swasthyakhabar.comw, accessed on 20/5/2019.

The Himalayan Times (2018) Around 200 nurses move out of TUTH in three years available online at: https://thehimalayantimes.com/nepal/around-200-nurses-move-tuth-three-years/, accessed on 27/4/2019.

Tschudin, V. & A.J. Davis (2008) *The globalisation of nursing*. Radcliffe Publishing, Abingdon.

TUTH (Tribhuwan University Teaching Hospital) (2018) Vacancies for staff nurses at Thribhuwan University Teaching Hospital (TUTH), available online at: https://

edusanjal.com/vacancy/tu-teaching-hospital-exam-control-division-announced-va cancy-staff-nurse/, accessed on 20/6/2019.

UNIFEM (United Nations Development Fund for Women) & NIDS (Nepal Institute of Development Studies) (2006) *Nepali women and foreign labour migration.* UNIFEM, New York and NIDS, Kathmandu.

Waters, A. (2010) The question for universities: how can they win the war on attrition? *Nursing Standard*, 24(24): 12–15.

Winkelmann-Gleed, A. (2006) *Migrant nurses: motivation, integration and contribution.* Radcliffe Publishing, Abingdon.

Wojczewski, S., A. Poppe, K. Hoffmann, W. Peersmann, O. Nka, S. Pentz, & R. Kutale Omazana (2015) Diaspora engagement of African migrant health workers: examples from five destination countries, *Global Health Action*, available online at: www.ncbi.nlm.nih.gov/pmc/articles/PMC4676361/, accessed on 20/2/2019.

WHO (World Health Organisation) (2006) *Working together for health: the World Health Report*, available online at: www.who.int/whr/2006/en/, accessed on 20/6/2019.

Yeate's, N. (2008) Here to stay? Migrant health workers in Ireland. In J. Connell (ed.) *The international migration of health workers*, pp. 62–76. Routledge, Abingdon.

Zimmerman, M., R. Shakya, B.M. Pokhrel, N. Eyal, B.P. Rijal, R.N. Shrestha, & A. Syami (2012) Medical students' characteristics as predictors of career practice location: retrospective cohort study tracking graduates of Nepal's first medical college, *BMJ*, 345. https://doi.org/10.1136/bmj.e4826.

Zimmerman, M.K., J.S. Litt, & C.E. Bose (2006) *Global dimensions of gender and carework.* Stanford University Press, Stanford, CA.

Index

Printed in the United States
by Baker & Taylor Publisher Services